HISTORY
OF THE
CONGRESS
OF
NEUROLOGICAL
SURGEONS
1951-1991

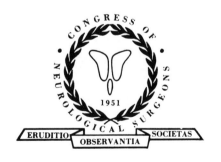

HISTORY
OF THE
CONGRESS
OF
NEUROLOGICAL
SURGEONS
1951-1991

Editor

JOHN M. THOMPSON, MD

Historian and Chairman

Archives Committee

Sponsored by the Congress of Neurological Surgeons

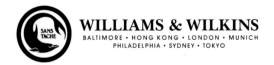

WILLIAMS & WILKINS
BALTIMORE · HONG KONG · LONDON · MUNICH
PHILADELPHIA · SYDNEY · TOKYO

Printed in the United States of America

Library of Congress
Catalog Card Number
00-00000
ISBN 0-683-08181-0

The History of the Congress of Neurological Surgeons, 1951–1991 / editor, John M. Thompson : sponsored by the Congress of Neurological Surgeons.
    p.   cm.
  ISBN 0-683-08181-0
  1. Neurosurgeons—United States—Biography. 2. Congress of Neurological Surgeons—History. I. Thompson, John M. (John Morgan), 1924– . II. Congress of Neurological Surgeons.
  [DNLM: 1. Congress of Neurological Surgeons.
  2. Neurosurgery—United States—societies.   3. Societies, Medical—history—United States.   WL 1 C749h]
  RD592.8.H57   1991
  617.4′8′006073—dc20
  DNLM/DLC
  for Library of Congress   91-30725
                                                          CIP

Preface

May 11, 1991 was the 40th birthday of the Congress of Neurological Surgeons (CNS). On that date in 1951, 22 young neurosurgeons met in St. Louis, Missouri and founded the Congress of Neurological Surgeons. For the past several years, the Executive Committee of the CNS has been planning a volume on the history of the CNS. Dr. Michael Salcman, current CNS president, felt that it would be appropriate to publish a commemorative history in our 40th year. He subsequently asked me to assemble the biographies of all our honored guests and presidents. I insisted that this volume also include his biography and the biography of this year's honored guest, Dr. Bennett Stein. The biographies of our past honored guests, starting with the 1956 volume containing the biography of Dr. Wilder G. Penfield, are reprinted from *Clinical Neurosurgery* with some modifications. Dr. Stephen W. Papadopoulous kindly prepared a biography of our first honored guest, Dr. Herbert Olivecrona. I prepared the biography of our second honored guest, Sir Geoffrey Jefferson, using material from the obituary published in Volume 18 of the *Journal of Neurosurgery*. This obituary was written by Dr. E. Harry Botterell. A biography of our third honored guest, Dr. Kenneth G. McKenzie, was prepared by one of our outstanding Canadian neurosurgeons, Dr. Thomas P. Morley and the biography of our fourth honored guest, Dr. Carl W. Rand, was prepared by his son, Dr. Robert Rand, a distinguished neurosurgeon in Los Angeles. Three of our past presidents are deceased. The biography of Dr. Elmer S. Schultz was prepared by Dr. Richard DeSaussure, Jr. of Memphis. The biography of Dr. Hendrick J. Svien was prepared by Dr. Nayef Al-Rodham, a resident in neurological surgery at the Mayo Clinic. The biography of Dr. Donald B. Sweeney was prepared by his son, Mr. Donald Sweeney, Jr., an attorney in Birmingham, Alabama.

This history is obviously incomplete in that it does not contain biographies of many neurosurgeons who have made major contributions to our profession and it does not contain the biographies of many members of the CNS who devoted their talents and time to make this organization one of the largest and best neurosurgical societies in the world. I cannot speak for other years, but I can say that in 1970 the strongest and the best neurosurgeons in the CNS were on the bottom of the pyramid while I was a lightweight on top.

I have attended every meeting of the Congress of Neurological Surgeons since the 1958 meeting in San Francisco and have found every meeting intellectually stimulating and socially delightful. I am not a founding member and I owe a great debt of gratitude to several founding members who have helped me greatly in preparing the history of the early years of the Congress. In 1970, when I was President, Dr. Bland Cannon, the first secretary and the sixth president of the CNS, sent me all his historical material. I used his historical material to prepare my presidential address. Dr. James R. Gay, the fourth president of the CNS, also sent me much information about the founding and early years of the Congress. Dr. Richard DeSaussure was the first historian and he sent the archives to me at the time I became historian and chairman of the Archives Committee. Dr. DeSaussure has been most cooperative. Dr. A. Roy Tyrer has also provided much valuable historical material.

The Congress has had a superb relationship with Williams & Wilkins for the past 36 years. I would like to express my appreciation to Carol-Lynn Brown and Anne Stewart Seitz of Williams & Wilkins, for their assistance.

Last, but not least, I would like to express my appreciation to Dorothy, my office nurse, my secretary, my friend, and my wife who has been my partner in all of my Congress endeavors including this one. She typed much of this manuscript and her support has been invaluable.

JOHN M. THOMPSON, M.D.
HISTORIAN AND CHAIRMAN, ARCHIVES COMMITTEE
CONGRESS OF NEUROLOGICAL SURGEONS

Founding Members

F.S. Barringer
Leon M. Becker
Carrol A. Brown
Bland W. Cannon
Richard L. DeSaussure
John W. Devanney
Franklin Earnest, III
Edward M. Gates
James R. Gay
Philip D. Gordy
Warren C. Hastings

John A. Hetherington
Nathaniel R. Hollister
Donathan Ivey
Thomas M. Marshall
F.A. Palazzo
Frederick C. Rehfeldt
Elmer C. Schultz
H.J. Svien
Donald B. Sweeney
A. Roy Tyrer
Edgar N. Weaver

Distinguished Service Award Winners

Lycurgus M. Davey–1966
Walter S. Lockhart, Jr.–1969
Edward J. Bishop–1970
George Ablin–1971
William S. Coxe–1973
J.F. Ross Fleming–1975
Perry Black–1977
William A. Buchheit–1979

Edwin Amyes–1980
Edward F. Downing–1984
J. Charles Rich–1986
Ronald I. Apfelbaum–1987
E. Fletcher Eyster–1988
Fremont P. Wirth–1989
Merwyn Bagan–1990

CNS Resident Award Winners

Arthur I. Kobrine–1974
Stephen Brem–1975
Philip H. Gutin–1976
Robert F. Spetzler–1977
Martin G. Luken, III–1978
George R. Prioleau–1979
Larry V. Carson–1980
Ted S. Keller–1981
Mervin P. Kril–1982

J.F. Graham–1983
Fredric Meyer–1984
Emily D. Friedman–1985
Victoria C. Neave–1986
Lew Disney–1987
Martin E. Weinand–1988
Nayef R.F. Al-Rodhan–1989
Ivar Mendez–1990

CNS Clinical Fellowship Award Winners

Brian Andrews–1987
Charles Branch–1987
Randall Powell–1987
Eric Zager–1988
Jonathan Hodes–1989

James Rutka–1989
Claudio Feler–1990
Mazen Khayata–1990
Prem Pillay–1991

Introduction

The birth certificate of neurological surgery in the United States was issued on November 18, 1904 when Dr. Harvey Cushing presented a paper at the Academy of Medicine in Cleveland with the title, "The Special Field of Neurological Surgery." Neurology was already a well-recognized specialty and the American Neurological Association had been founded in 1874. In March 1920, the Society of Neurological Surgeons was founded by 11 neurosurgeons attending a meeting in Boston. The number of neurosurgeons gradually increased, and many of these younger neurosurgeons keenly wanted professional contact with their neurosurgical colleagues in order to increase their knowledge and to keep up with the rapid advances in their specialty. The Society of Neurological Surgeons had, however, limited its membership and many of the younger neurosurgeons were not invited to join. As a result, on October 10, 1931 Drs. Temple Fay, Eustance Semmes, Glen Spurling, and W. E. Van Wagenen met in Washington, DC to plan a new society. Dr. Fay suggested the name "Harvey Cushing Society" after Dr. Cushing expressed his approval of the new group. Thirty charter members were chosen and the Harvey Cushing Society had its first meeting in Boston on May 6, 1932. Membership initially was limited to 35 as it was felt that a small group was desirable in order to allow an exchange of ideas. It is of interest to note that, when he welcomed the Society to his clinic, Dr. Cushing remarked that in another 10 years another neurosurgical group would be formed which would look upon the members of the Harvey Cushing Society as senile and antiquated. Dr. Cushing's prediction proved to be somewhat conservative, as in 1938 seven young neurosurgeons who had not been elected into the Harvey Cushing Society met in Memphis, Tennessee and organized the American Academy of Neurological Surgery. The Academy vowed to keep its doors open to newcomers, but the need for close fellowship and education eventually caused this group, too, to restrict membership.

Major changes in neurological surgery took place in the 1940s. Before that, only relatively small numbers of neurosurgeons completed training each year. World War II, however, had a marked impact on medicine and particularly on neurological surgery. Medical education was accelerated so that medical schools were turning out graduates in 3 rather than 4 years. Internships were reduced from 1 year to 9 months. Most young physicians joined the armed forces before completing their residency training and many developed their surgical skills helping to care for the enormous numbers of war casualties. Most of these men matured far more rapidly than they might have with an equal number of years experience in civilian life. Many of these young surgeons were assigned to neurosurgical units where they developed an interest in the specialty under the tutelage of experienced neurosurgeons. After their release from active duty, these mature but young and partially trained surgeons applied for civilian residencies. Grateful and patriotic program directors accepted many more people into their programs than they had previously been accustomed to training. Although the American Board of Neurological Surgery, which was founded in 1940, required only 2 years of neurosurgical residency training, few men completed their training in less than 6 or 7 postgraduate years.

Before World War II, most neurological surgeons were associated with academic centers where there were opportunities to discuss problem cases with colleagues. Many young neurological surgeons completing their training, however, went into solo private practice in areas that had not previously had neurosurgeons. These young men soon felt the need for continuing education and to belong to a national group of neurological surgeons. After 1948, the number of neurological surgeons completing training rapidly increased and the existing national neurosurgical societies were reluctant to expand their memberships to accommodate this growth. In June 1948, the Neurological Society of America was established in Chicago, but this group also chose to limit its membership. The Harvey Cushing Society, which by 1949 had opened up its membership and had expanded into an organization of national scope with 148 members, would not admit members until they were Board Certified. The Board, however, had a waiting period of at least 2 years after completing training before a young neurosurgeon could take the examination. Therefore, the lag time between completing training and being accepted into membership in the Harvey Cushing Society was *at least* 3 years. Thus the stage was set for the establishment of another national neurosurgical society.

In September 1950, several neurosurgeons met at Sea Island, Georgia and discussed the possibility of forming a new national society. This discussion continued in February 1951 at the meeting of the Southern Neurosurgical Society in New Orleans. Just after the conclusion of the Interurban Neurosurgical Society meeting in Chicago, nine neurological surgeons met in a room at the Palmer House on February 24, 1951 to discuss in more detail the formation of the new society. This meeting was attended by Drs. Floyd S. Barringer, Bland W. Cannon, James R. Gay, Louis J. Gogela, Nathaniel R. Hollister, Wiber A. Muehlig, David B. Roth, Elmer C. Schultz, and Emil P. Phelan. Dr. Cannon was appointed chairman *pro tem* and Dr. Gay was appointed secretary *pro tem*. This group decided to hold an organizational meeting on May 10, 1951, just after the examination of the American Board of Neurological Surgery. Letters were sent out to approximately 50 neurosurgeons inviting their suggestions about the formation of a new neurosurgical society. This letter explained that the proposed new group had no intention of competing with the existing societies.

On May 11, 1951, 22 young neurosurgeons met at the Jefferson Hotel in St. Louis, Missouri to found this new neurosurgical society. The name "Congress of Neurological Surgeons" was selected with care. "American" was deliberately not used as the founders wanted the new organization to be international with unlimited membership, concepts that formed the base for the new society's constitution. It was also recognized that the initials CNS were the abbreviation commonly used for the central nervous system, the target for many neurosurgical operations. The Congress would be an association of neurosurgeons organized to study and discuss the principles of neurological surgery, to study developments in scientific fields allied to neurosurgery, and to honor living leaders in the field of neurosurgery. The founders recognized that there were very few honors in neurosurgery commensurate with the difficulty of becoming a respected member of that fraternity. To correct this shortcoming, the Congress introduced the practice of honoring a world-class neurosurgeon at the annual meeting.

At the time of the founding meeting in St. Louis, Dr. Elmer C. Schultz was elected president, Dr. Carrol A. Brown was elected vice president, and Dr. Bland W. Cannon was elected secretary. It was decided that the first scientific meeting would be held in Memphis, Tennessee. Committees were appointed and the enthusiastic members of the Congress worked long and hard to ensure the success of their first annual meeting. The 11 members of the Steering Committee were asked to donate $50.00 each to the Congress to provide funds to meet expenses until the time of the first annual meeting. The members of the Congress will forever owe a debt of gratitude to these men for subsidizing the organization in such a critical period in its history. The annual dues of the Congress were set at $25.00 and were not increased for 20 years.

The founding members of the CNS had many unique talents. Dr. Hank Svien became the national strategist, putting out fires started by older neurosurgeons. Dr. Bland Cannon was the internal strategist, selling ideas to the members and proposing candidates for membership. Dr. Jim Gay was the logistics person, planner, and organizer.

By August 1951 the Congress had 69 members and was already an international organization with active members from the United States, Canada, Mexico, Chile, and Cuba. The first annual meeting of the Congress was held at the Peabody Hotel in Memphis, Tennessee from Thursday, November 15 to Saturday, November 17, 1951 and was attended by 63 of its 121 members, 17 guests, and nine guest speakers. The legal advisor, Mr. Dunlap Cannon, Jr. prepared the Charter for the Congress and the Congress was incorporated in the State of Tennessee on November 15, 1951. A review of the schedule of fees to this meeting reveals the extent of inflation that has taken place since 1951. Luncheon tickets sold for $2.50 per person and banquet tickets were $5.00.

A Ladies Auxiliary was organized at the meeting in Memphis. Before then neurosurgical meetings were "bachelor" affairs. CNS leaders were sensitive to the loneliness spouses faced as a result of erratic schedules and long hours. It was thought that a bachelor meeting out of town only aggravated the problem. Therefore, spouses were encouraged to attend and to engage in an interesting program of their own. This policy resulted in making the annual meeting much more fun for everyone. There was less shop talk and more rest for everyone. The annual meeting became an important social event as well as a needed professional experience. The Auxiliary of the Congress of Neurological Surgeons has continued to play a very important part in the Congress and many spouses have worked side-by-side with their neurosurgeons in Congress activities.

The Executive Committee authorized publication of the *Congress Newsletter* in February 1952. Dr. Roy Tyrer was appointed the first editor. In November 1953, the Executive Committee authorized publication of *Clinical Neurosurgery*. Dr. Raymond K. Thompson was the first editor-in-chief. Following the 1953 meeting in New Orleans there was the first post-convention tour under the direction of Jorge Picaza. The Congress seal was officially adopted in November 1954.

In June 1956, the Executive Committee authorized the chairman of the Survey Committee, Dr. John R. Russell, to publish a *Directory of Neurological Surgeons in the United States*. In 1966 and 1967 the Congress published its first *World Directory of Neurological Surgeons* with Dr. George Ablin as editor.

In 1966, the Socio-Economics Committee of the Congress under the chairmanship of Edward Bishop, published *The Tabulation of the Results of a National Fee Survey*. The Utilization Guidelines Committee, under the chairmanship of Dr. Walter S. Lockhart, Jr., prepared a manual, *Neurosurgical Utilization Guidelines*, which was published by the Congress in 1969.

The Congress has always been very interested in neurosurgical residents and on May 19, 1958, the Executive Committee authorized the expenditure of Congress funds to provide free lodging for residents attending the annual meeting.

The Congress was founded as an international neurosurgical society and its history in that arena is impressive. The Congress actively supported the formation of the Foundation for International Education in Neurological Surgery. The Congress is a member society of the World Federation of Neurosurgical Societies and participates actively in its international congresses.

In 1972, the Executive Committee studied the feasibility of establishing its own neurosurgical journal and then authorized the publication of *Neurosurgery*. The journal was first published in 1977 with Robert H. Wilkins as its first editor. Four volumes of *Concepts in Neurosurgery* have now been published under the direction of Drs. Fremont P. Wirth and Robert A. Ratcheson. These volumes cover a specific area in depth with basic scientific knowledge and theory applied to practical neurosurgical issues. *Clinical Neurosurgery* continues to be published with Volume 38 available this year.

The Congress of Neurological Surgeons has become one of the largest neurosurgical societies in the world. At the time of our twentieth anniversary meeting in St. Louis, the Congress had 1,260 members in all 50 States, seven Canadian provinces, and 28 other nations on every continent except Antarctica. At the present time the Congress has 3,636 members, including 615 residents and 243 international members.

Contents

1961: NEW YORK

1962: HOUSTON

1963: DENVER

1964: MIAMI

1965: CHICAGO

1966: SAN JUAN

1967: SAN FRANCISCO

1968: TORONTO

1969: BOSTON

1970: ST. LOUIS

1971: MIAMI

1972: DENVER

1973: HONOLULU

1974: VANCOUVER

1975: ATLANTA

1976: NEW ORLEANS

1977: SAN FRANCISCO

1978: WASHINGTON, DC

1979: LAS VEGAS

1980: HOUSTON

1981: LOS ANGELES

1982: TORONTO

1983: CHICAGO

1984: NEW YORK

xviCONTENTS

1951

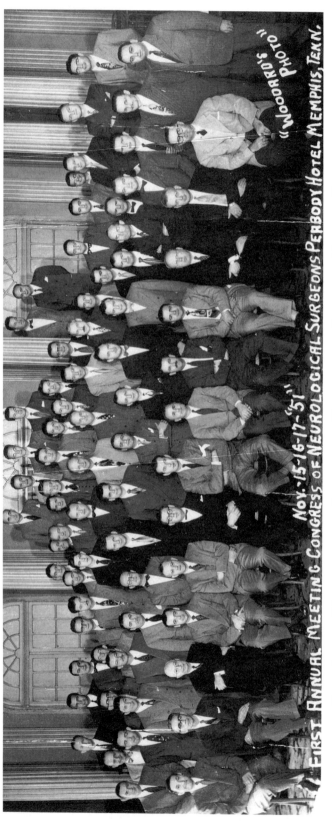

First Annual Meeting of the Congress of Neurological Surgeons, Memphis, Tennessee

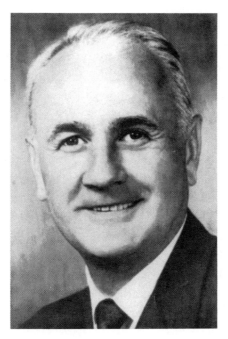

Elmer C. Schultz

Elmer C. Schultz, "Dutch" as he was known to his many friends, was born and raised in Michigan. He received his medical degree from the University of Michigan, and took part of his neurosurgical training at the Henry Ford Hospital. During World War II, he served in a neurosurgical unit stationed in England. Dr. Glen Spurling was the neurosurgical consultant and frequently called the neurosurgeons serving in England to conferences in London. Dr. Schultz developed his expertise with peripheral nerves during this time.

After World War II, Dr. Schultz completed his training at the University of Virginia under Dr. Gayle Crutchfield. After completing his training, he remained at the University of Virginia for 1 year as an instructor.

In 1948 Dr. Schultz was invited to join Drs. Semmes and Murphey in Memphis and was a productive member of the Semmes-Murphey Clinic until his untimely death in 1967 at the age of 55. He had acquired a peculiar type of arthritis with fibrosis of his lungs. Dr. Schultz was a founding member of the Congress of Neurological Surgeons and served as its first president when this young organization met in Memphis in 1951.

Dr. Schultz and his wife, Marge, had one son and three daughters. One of his daughters graduated from nursing school and performed her duties in an excellent manner at the Baptist Memorial Hospital where her father carried out his neurosurgical practice. Dr. Schultz took up flying late in his career, and felt the happiest when he was carrying out a neurosurgical procedure or flying his plane.

RICHARD DeSAUSSURE, JR., M.D.

1952

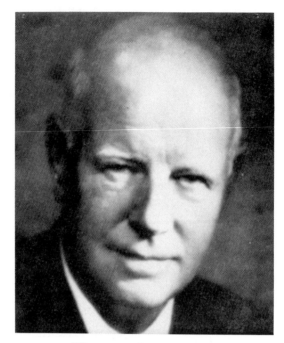

HERBERT OLIVECRONA

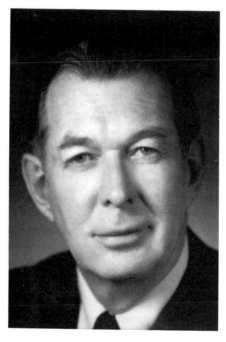

HENDRIK JULIUS SVIEN

Herbert Olivecrona

Herbert Olivecrona began his brilliant career in the surgical department of Serafimer Hospital. He established the first neurosurgery department at that hospital in 1930. In 1935, he was appointed professor of neurosurgery at the Karolinska Institute, a post he held until his retirement in 1960. He was a member of the Swedish Academy of Science and numerous Scandinavian, European, and American medical and surgical societies. He was a champion of international scholarship, sparked by a year he spent as a young man in 1919 at The Johns Hopkins Hospital in Baltimore. Harvey Cushing planted the seed of neurosurgical interest in the young Dr. Olivecrona. Cushing offered him a year's residency, but Dr. Olivecrona was unable to finance the year abroad.

During the 1920s Herbert Olivecrona single-handedly established the neurosurgical program at Serafimer Hospital and became a contemporary expert in brain tumor surgery. Shortly thereafter he embarked on his career at the Karolinska Institute for which he is most recognized. One of his earliest collaborators was Eric Lysholm, the Swedish radiologist who developed the art of pneumoencephalography. Eric Lindgren later became Dr. Olivecrona's radiologist and Dr. Lindgren's work helped neuroradiology become a distinct and respected subspecialty. Dr. Olivecrona's disciples are equally known and respected in the international community and include Lars Leksell, Gosta Norlen, Olath Sjoqvist, Einar Bohm, and Eduard Busch.

Dr. Olivecrona was not satisfied merely to operate with low surgical mortality. His aim was always to restore his patients to good functional condition and to cure them whenever possible. He was one of the first to save the facial nerve in operations for removal of acoustic neuromas and gradually improved his results until he was able to save the nerve function in 65% of the cases in which he operated. He was also an adept and skilled cerebrovascular surgeon, contributing much to the current understanding and care of patients with cerebral aneurysms and arteriovenous malfunctions. Herbert Olivecrona was probably the first to realize that competent anesthesia in neurosurgery could only be obtained by having a specialized neuroanesthesiologist, and he found one in Emerick Gordon.

Herbert Olivecrona's unique prominence for so many decades can be comprehended fully only if his achievements are viewed in the appropriate historical perspective. Until the early 1920s, when he began neurosurgery, the diagnosis of a brain tumor was equivalent to a death sentence. Neurosurgery had only begun to make its first faltering steps.

Dr. Olivecrona traveled widely, observed others, and synthesized their insights. At the same time he developed his own neurosurgical techniques and principles, bringing about giant steps of progress in the field. In the annals of international neurosurgery, he is remembered with a reverence similar to that reserved for Harvey Cushing and Walter Dandy. Herbert Olivecrona died in January 1980.

STEPHEN M. PAPADOPOULOUS, M.D.

Hendrik Julius Svien

Hendrik (Hank) Julius Svien was born in a farming community near Rochester, Minnesota, of Norwegian parentage in 1911. He entered St. Olaf College and graduated *cum laude* in chemistry. He later undertook graduate work in chemistry at the Massachusetts Institute of Technology and a teaching appointment at New York University. He abandoned chemistry to enter the University of Minnesota Medical School and earned an M.D. degree in 1937. In 1938, he was appointed a fellow in general surgery at the Mayo Clinic and later in neurosurgery, and was "boarded" in both specialities.

Dr. Svien served in the United States Navy Medical Corps during World War II between 1942 and 1946. During this period, he was stationed at Portsmouth, Bethesda, the Fleet Marine Force, and at Oceanside, advancing in rank to lieutenant commander and was awarded three battle stars. He met his future wife, Nancy Weems Gatch (the daughter of Admiral and Mrs. Thomas Leigh Gatch) while on active duty. He returned to the Mayo Clinic in 1948, where he remained on staff in the Department of Neurological Surgery until his untimely death in 1972.

Dr. Svien had a keen interest in research and in a wide range of clinical problems. He participated in the development of a new classification of glial tumors with Drs. Kernohan, Mabon, Adson, and Craig. He had an interest in the surgical treatment of torticollis, pituitary tumors, malignant brain lesions, and cerebral edema. He investigated the use of steroids in animals with cerebral edema before its application in humans by Dr. Lyle French. He described with Dr. Hollenhorst, a method to measure retinal artery pressure and explained its importance.

Dr. Svien was founder and second president of the Congress of Neurological Surgeons. He served on the Board of Directors of the American Association of Neurological Surgeons and as secretary and treasurer. He became a member of all the national neurosurgical organizations and was chairman of the Foundation for International Education in Neurosurgery.

Dr. Svien published more than 120 articles, as well as one book on the treatment of pituitary tumors, and died in 1972 from congestive heart failure. He is remembered by those who knew him as a talented investigator and surgeon.

NAYEF R. F. AL-RODHAN, M.D., PH.D.

1953

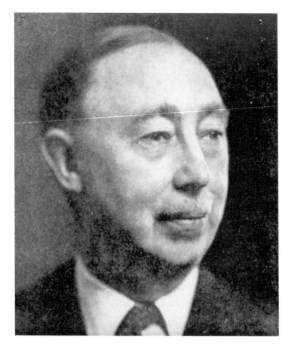

SIR GEOFFREY JEFFERSON

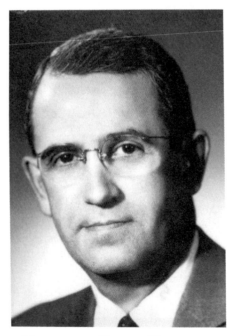

NATHANIEL ROGER HOLLISTER

Sir Geoffrey Jefferson

Sir Geoffrey Jefferson was born April 10, 1886. His father was a general practitioner and surgeon. Jefferson studied medicine at the University of Manchester and graduated with honors. He received his house officer training in Manchester and in London. He joined the Royal Army Medical Corps and was assigned in 1915 to the Anglo-Russian Hospital in St. Petersburg, Russia. He was there at the time of the Revolution. He then was transferred to the 14th General Hospital in France.

After World War I, Jefferson visited Harvey Cushing in Boston. He became the first neurosurgeon at the Manchester Royal Infirmary in 1926 but had only four beds at his disposal. He received an invitation in 1933 to join the staff of the National Hospital in Queens Square and visited London every two weeks to consult and to operate. Manchester University created the first chairmanship of neurological surgery in 1939 and named Sir Geoffrey Jefferson as the first professor. He was primarily responsible for the founding of the Society of British Neurological Surgeons.

Jefferson treated many of the British neurosurgical casualties in World War II and he was honored by appointment as a Commander of the Order of the British Empire in 1943. He was elected a Fellow of the Royal Society in 1947 and was knighted in 1950.

Sir Geoffrey Jefferson made major contributions to the treatment of head and spinal injuries. He also had a particular interest in pituitary adenomas and saccular aneurysms.

Sir Geoffrey Jefferson was the second honored guest of the Congress in 1953 in New Orleans and became president of the first International Congress of Neurological Surgeons in Brussels in 1957. Sir Geoffrey's papers for the Congress meeting concerned changing views on the integration of the brain, trigeminal neuromas, and compression of the optic pathways by intracranial aneurysms.

Jefferson married Gertrude Flumerfelt of Victoria, British Columbia in 1914. The Jeffersons had 3 children, Dr. Michael Jefferson, Mr. Anthony Jefferson, and Lady Monical Bruce Gardner. Sir Geoffrey Jefferson died on January 20, 1961 at the age of 74.

Nathaniel Roger Hollister

Nathaniel Roger Hollister was born on May 18, 1915. He was the third son of Robert R. Hollister, M.D. and Susan Holdredge. Dr. Hollister stood in considerable awe of his physician father and seldom directly opposed his wishes. His father discouraged medicine as a career and he recommended that his three sons do something together as a team. Dr. Hollister's two older brothers were scholastic achievers and feeling he was not, Dr. Hollister did not relish life in the shadow of his two older brothers. He attended Antioch College and requested that his Antioch cooperative job be in New York City. He was willing to take any job in New York City and subsequently found himself at the New York Hospital-Cornell University Medical Center. That job convinced Na-

thaniel Hollister that he wanted to be a physician. He enrolled in and graduated from the University of Nebraska School of Medicine. Postgraduate training
was obtained at the Boston City Hospital. He became very interested in neurological surgery and started his training at the Massachusetts General Hospital and then had two additional years of training with Dr. Jefferson Browder
at the Kings County Hospital.

Dr. Hollister served as a neurosurgeon during World War II and had the
incredible experience of "cleaning up" one of the notorious concentration camps.
After he was discharged from military service, Dr. Hollister became a staff
neurosurgeon at the Oschner Clinic. He later entered private practice in Dayton, Ohio. There were no neurologists in Dayton, so Dr. Hollister practiced
both neurology and neurosurgery. The Dayton area served 500,000 people so
he was quite busy. Dr. Hollister desperately wanted a neurosurgical organization to relieve the isolation of private practice and to promote the education
of and contact between neurosurgeons. Nathaniel Hollister, Bland Cannon,
Elmer Schultz, Jim Gay, Don Sweeney, and Hank Svien wrote letters to all
the young neurosurgeons that they knew who had entered practice after the
conclusion of World War II. Dr. Hollister was one of 22 men who gathered in
St. Louis on May 11, 1951 to found the Congress of Neurological Surgeons.
Dr. Hollister became president of the Congress in 1953 when the meeting was
held in New Orleans.

Dr. Hollister remembers well the last presentation of the honored guest at
the 1953 meeting, Sir Geoffrey Jefferson. He recalled that Sir Geoffrey Jefferson concluded his last presentation with a few off-the-cuff remarks. These
were, "Of course you know that, really, the glamour has gone out of neurosurgery. You boys aren't where you were. The heart people have stolen it from
you. Well, my answer to that is if any branch of surgery is doing work which
is in any way comparable to our own, we welcome that development. We have
grown up and in time they will do so, too." Dr. Hollister has been thinking
about that quote ever since.

Dr. Hollister became very interested in pain and noted that even though
neurological surgeons could technically attack the pain paradox, the results
were frequently not satisfactory. Dr. Hollister felt that in order to deal more
adequately with complicated pain problems he needed additional training. He
had been previously Board certified in neurological surgery and with additional
training he became Board certified in neurology and psychiatry. Dr. Hollister
established the Boston Pain Unit in 1972 and felt that was one of his more
gratifying accomplishments. He demonstrated that chronic pain suffering is a
"learned behavior" that can be changed.

1954

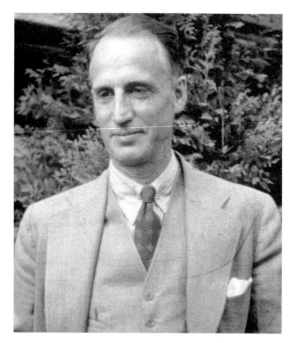

KENNETH GEORGE McKENZIE

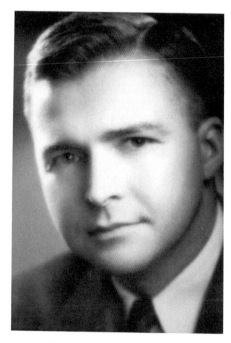

JAMES ROWLAND GAY

Kenneth George McKenzie

After his return from the trenches on the western front in World War I, Kenneth G. McKenzie set up a general practice in Toronto to support his wife and young family. As soon as the opportunity came his way he accepted an offer as house surgeon to Harvey Cushing in Boston, which led to his appointment as neurosurgeon at the Toronto General Hospital and the University of Toronto.

His was the first neurosurgical appointment in Canada. Dr. McKenzie used to say, somewhat mischievously, that it wasn't until Professor Archibald, McGill's professor of surgery, saw him perform a selective trigeminal rhizotomy for tic douloureux by the middle fossa approach that Archibald decided it was time Montreal had a neurosurgeon. The result of this decision was the appointment of Wilder Penfield to McGill's medical faculty and the founding of the famous Montreal Neurological Institute.

Dr. McKenzie's father, Alexander F. McKenzie, practiced medicine in the village of Monkton, Ontario, where Kenneth attended primary school. Medicine must have been a natural career choice for the only son of a practitioner who became, according to the *Alameda Times Star* of 4 October 1951, the "oldest practicing physician in the British Empire," and who, "on the occasion of his 65th year of practice last year ... was signally honoured by his colleagues, by the King and Queen, and by the Lieutenant Governor (*sic*) of Canada." (This was a misprint for Governor General.)

In 1905, Kenneth graduated from elementary school in Monkton and was accepted into St. Andrew's College, which was then in Toronto. He eventually earned a First in General Proficiency and Second Class Honours. In his final year he played on the 2nd rugby team and the 1st cricket XI. He was beaten in the featherweight (115 lbs) boxing division but won at wrestling. The school's reputation in wrestling was at its peak in those years. In 1908 "Dutch" Bollard was the "the youngest schoolboy ever to achieve so great a success as coming second in the Canadian Wrestling Championship." McKenzie carried his athletic ability to the University of Toronto where he was captain of the senior medical rugby team the year it won the Mulock Cup, and he became intercollegiate bantam weight wrestling champion in his second year.

The photograph reproduced here was taken when he was at the zenith of his neurosurgical career. It gives the clear impression of modest amiability. What it conceals is his ruthless application to the mastery of a skill, whether professional or recreational. He was driven by a flair for invention and a compulsion for perfection. He practiced his golf swing by tirelessly beating golf balls by the bucketful against a net he had erected on his lawn at home. He attempted to analyze his swing by monitoring the pitch of a whistling device attached to the head of the club. He earned a place on the Canadian Seniors' golf team. He was no less dedicated to the pursuit of perfection in salmon fishing.

These personal qualities attracted neurosurgical trainees to whom Dr. McKenzie was a patient and very personal teacher. The first generation of Canadian neurosurgeons came from his stable. He was very much a part of that early band of brothers who were the American neurosurgeons between the First and Second World Wars.

In his neurosurgical writings Dr. McKenzie held to the disciplined surgical line and avoided, even in later life, artless diversions and ruminations on his career and days gone by. Apart from solid reports of the results of treatment in acoustic neuroma, intracranial abscess, glioma, lumbar disc, and other conditions, his originality was demonstrated in articles on the treatment of spasmodic torticollis by intradural division of the spinal roots of the 11th nerve and roots of the upper cervical nerve (1924, 1955), the mechanics of paraplegia and its surgical relief in non-neoplastic scoliosis (1927, 1949), the surgical treatment of tic douloureux (1925, 1933), intracranial division of the vestibular portion of the 8th nerve for intractable vertigo (1932, 1936, 1955), the results of frontal lobotomy in the treatment of mental disease (1946, 1954, 1964) and trigeminal medullary tractotomy (1955). He wrote short articles to demonstrate his designs of a leucotome for lobotomy, skull calipers for use in fractures of the cervical spine (with prompt acknowledgement, as soon as he became aware of its need, to Dr. Crutchfield who, unknown to Dr. McKenzie, had preceded him in describing a similar caliper), perforator and burr for the hand-operated Hudson's brace, and a modification of the Cushing hemostatic clip.

He became, by consensus of those who worked with him, the most dexterous of brain surgeons. He was a magician, with economy of movement, sure of the next step, unfaltering and unflappable. These qualities were matched only by the admiration and affection he commanded among his residents.

Dr. McKenzie's death was as ordered and self-assured as his life. Having refused medicinal palliation in his last protracted illness, he decided the time had come to announce quietly to his family that he wouldn't be coming downstairs anymore, and three days later he died in February 1964.

T. P. MORLEY

James Rowland Gay

Dr. James Rowland Gay was born in Dunmore, Pennsylvania on June 23, 1914. He received a B.S. degree from The Virginia Polytechnic and State University (1935), and an M.D. degree from The Johns Hopkins University School of Medicine (1939). He served as a house officer in surgery and psychiatry at The Johns Hopkins Hospital (1939–1941). A fellowship in neurosurgery at The Mayo Foundation and Clinic was interrupted by World War II (1942–1946). He was assigned to medical staff positions in the United States Army, obtained the rank of major, and was decorated by the United States and French governments.

During his postgraduate education at the Mayo Foundation and Clinic, Dr. Gay was certified in neurology by the American Board of Psychiatry and Neurology (1948) and received an M.S. degree in neurosurgery from The University of Minnesota (1949). Later he was certified in neurosurgery by the American Board of Neurological Surgery (1951).

Dr. Gay was engaged in the private practice of neurosurgery at Columbus, Ohio and Bethlehem, Pennsylvania (1949–1961), until his appointment as head of the Section on Neurological Surgery at the Lovelace Clinic, Albuquerque, New Mexico (1961–1968).

In Albuquerque his career was changed to full-time academic administration at the University of New Mexico School of Medicine, where he served as assistant dean for administration, organized the New Mexico Accident Investigation Program (studying automobile accident causation), and was director of the New Mexico Regional Medical Program (1968–1974).

Dr. Gay became associate vice president for health affairs at the University of Tennessee Center for the Health Sciences, Memphis, where he assisted in development of the central administrative structure, and was Director of International Programs with emphasis on Egypt and Japan (1974–1982).

Dr. Gay was a member of the strategy group that founded the Congress of Neurological Surgeons. His role was planner, organizer, and strategist. He promoted international affairs and assisted in the development of the World Federation of Neurosurgical Societies.

During his term as president (1954), he designed and standardized the annual meeting format and produced the *Annual Meeting Manual*, providing guidelines for future arrangements and program committees. A sophisticated exhibit program was added for the first time, and the technique of planned spontaneity for audience participation was introduced.

After retiring from the University of Tennessee (1982), he moved to Northeast Pennsylvania where he is a Board member and chairman of the Strategy Committee of Wayne Memorial Hospital, Honesdale, Pennsylvania. Dr. Gay and his wife Lillian enjoy an outdoor life on a private lake, fishing, hiking, and studying nature. He remembers his part in founding the Congress of Neurological Surgeons as his most memorable experience in professional life.

1955

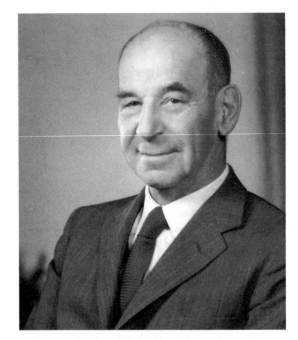

CARL WHEELER RAND

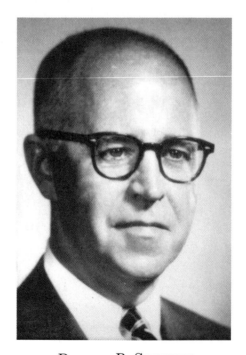

DONALD B. SWEENEY

Carl Wheeler Rand

Carl Wheeler Rand was born in Monson, Massachusetts on April 8, 1886, the son of Jenny Peck Rand and Nehemiah Wheeler Rand, a physician. Dr. Rand attended Monson Academy in Massachusetts and later Williams College from which he graduated in 1908 with a M.S. degree in English and as a member of Phi Beta Kappa.

In 1912, Dr. Rand graduated from The Johns Hopkins Medical School and did his internship under Dr. William Halstead. In 1913 he was the senior resident of Dr. John B. Murphy at Mercy Hospital in Chicago. He began his residency with Dr. Harvey Cushing on January 4, 1914 at Peter Bent Brigham Hospital in Boston.

Dr. Rand began his surgery practice in Los Angeles with Dr. Frederick Coller in 1916. This was interrupted in 1917 when he enlisted in the United States Army Medical Corps and went to France serving as a neurosurgeon near the front lines for 2 years. Upon returning to Los Angeles, Dr. Rand became chief of the staff of the Hospital of the Good Samaritan and the Los Angeles Children's Hospital. He started the neurological surgery services at the Los Angeles County General Hospital (University of Southern California Medical Center) as well as Wadsworth Veterans Administration Hospital and the Los Angeles Children's Hospital.

Dr. Rand was a member of the Society of Neurological Surgeons and served as its president in 1935. He was also a member of the American College of Surgeons, the Harvey Cushing Society, the Central Neuropsychiatric Association, the Los Angeles Academy of Medicine, the American Medical Association, the California Medical Society, and a diplomat of the American Board of Neurosurgery.

Dr. Rand was married to Katherine Humphrey and had three daughters and a son, Robert Rand, M.D. Dr. Carl Rand wrote more than 100 articles, three medical books, and a multitude of poems and songs.

ROBERT RAND, M.D.

Donald B. Sweeney

Dr. Donald B. Sweeney was born on March 17, 1917 in Mason City, Iowa. After receiving a B.S. degree from the University of Iowa he graduated from the University of Iowa College of Medicine in Iowa City in 1940. His house officer training was at Massachusetts General Hospital. He enlisted in the United States Army Medical Corps and served 18 months in the European Theatre as a captain with General Patton's army. He performed neurological surgery while in the Army.

Dr. Sweeney then returned to the Massachusetts General Hospital where he completed his neurosurgical training. He then went to the University of Iowa where he took additional training with Dr. Russell Meyers. He was invited to stay on the faculty of the University of Iowa and he remained there until 1953 when he moved to Birmingham, Alabama. He was an adjunct professor of neurological surgery at the University of Alabama School of Medicine. He practiced neurological surgery in Birmingham for many years. Dr. Sweeney was a founding member of the Congress of Neurological Surgeons and became the fifth president of the Congress, serving in 1955 when the Congress met in Los Angeles.

Dr. Sweeney was certified by the American Board of Neurological Surgery and was a member of the American Association of Neurological Surgeons, the American College of Surgeons, and the American Academy of Neurology. Dr. Sweeney and his wife Kathryn had four children. Mary K. Hight lives in Los Angeles; Donald B. Sweeney, Jr., an attorney, lives in Birmingham; Tandy H. Graves lives in Birmingham; and Alma Patricia Sears lives in Montevello, Alabama.

Dr. Sweeney died on March 7, 1982. Mrs. Sweeney now spends about 10 months each year in Bay Point, Florida and the other 2 months in Birmingham, Alabama.

DONALD B. SWEENEY, JR., J.D.

1956

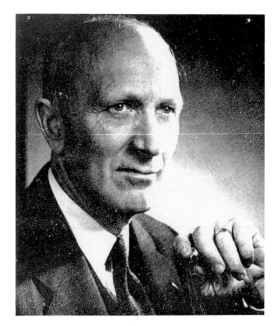

WILDER G. PENFIELD

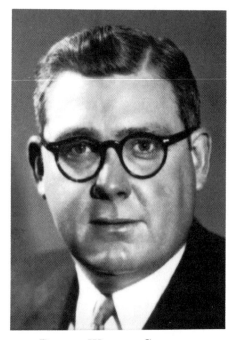

BLAND WILSON CANNON

Wilder G. Penfield

Dr. Penfield was a man of many facets. To the reader of this book an enumeration of his medical accomplishments would be redundant and therefore is omitted.

He was born in 1891, at Spokane, Washington, though since 1934 was a naturalized Canadian citizen. At Princeton University, he was an excellent student and a football star. He started one of the first Wilson for President Clubs on the Princeton Campus. In 1914 and 1919, he was a Rhodes scholar and has received three degrees from Oxford University. Interrupting his studies during the first World War, Dr. Penfield served in France the latter part of 1916 as a dresser and was wounded in 1917 while at sea aboard the S. S. Sussex. During his recuperation in England, he had the good fortune to convalesce at the home of Sir William and Lady Osler. The association with Sir William Osler exerted a great influence on our guest in the years that followed. After graduating from the Johns Hopkins Medical School in 1918 and spending several years in postgraduate study in Europe, he became associated with Columbia University and Presbyterian Hospital in New York. In 1928 he was selected to head the Department of Neurology and Neurosurgery at McGill University in Montreal. When the Rockefeller Foundation donated $1.25 million to McGill University to establish a Neurological Center to be second-to-none on this continent, it was understood that Dr. Penfield would be at its head.

He enjoyed membership in many societies—both on this continent and abroad. He was a Fellow of the Royal Society of London, the Royal College of Surgeons, the Royal College of Physicians, and the Royal Society of Medicine. He was also an Honorary Fellow of Merton College at Oxford.

Since 1939 he received 14 honorary degrees and was specially honored by having received the Order of Saint Michael and Saint George in 1943, the United States Medal of Freedom With Silver Palms in 1948, the Chevalier of Legion of Honor in 1950, and in 1953, the pinnacle of awards, the Order of Merit, conferred by Queen Elizabeth II. The Order of Merit is the highest honor that the Queen can confer upon her Commonwealth subjects and is limited to only 24 members. In 1954 he was elected to membership in the Athenaeum Club in London, which is reserved exclusively for men of great accomplishments in the Arts and Science.

Turning to the literary field in 1954, Dr. Penfield wrote "No Other Gods," a fictionalized version of Abraham's search for a monotheistic religion and his leadership of the Hebrew people on the journey to Canaan and a new destiny. When Dr. Penfield visited his mother in Los Angeles in 1935, she had completed a novel on the life of Sarah, wife of Abraham, leader of the Hebrew people. Since she appeared somewhat dissatisfied with her work he offered to take the manuscript with him and join her in authorship. However, she died a few months later. Nothing was done to this manuscript for the following 8 years. In 1943, during the War, Dr. Penfield was in Mesopotamia and read in a private library at Teheran an account of the excavation of Ur. Ten days later he crossed the desert to Ur and 11 years later completed his novel "No Other Gods." He twice visited the site of ancient Ur while writing his book and brought to the recreation of those ancient days the scientist's thoroughness. He also wrote a novel about Hippocrates and, with his usual thoroughness, visited the islands of Greece to obtain first-hand information.

As head of the Montreal Neurological Institute he was like a father, watching and guiding his large international family. Both he and Mrs. Penfield gave each new Fellow, no matter what part of the world he came from, a feeling of belonging. They shared Sundays and holidays—especially Christmas—with the Fellows in the Penfield home, along with their own children.

In conclusion, it is apropos to quote the president of Princeton in conferring on him an honorary degree—"A strong and gentle man with extraordinary dexterity." Dr. Penfield died in April 1976.

IRA J. JACKSON, M.D.

Bland Wilson Cannon

Bland Wilson Cannon was born on April 4, 1920 in Brownsville, Tennessee. He attended Rhodes College and received a B.S. degree in 1941. He then attended Northwestern University Graduate School and had a fellowship at the Institute of Neurology in 1942 and 1944. He received his M.D. degree from Northwestern University Medical School and interned at New York Hospital in New York City between 1944 and 1945. He had a fellowship at the Mayo Foundation from 1945 to 1946 and served as a captain in the Army Medical Corps at the 98th General Hospital in Germany from 1946 to 1948. He then returned to the Mayo Clinic in Rochester where he completed his neurosurgical training between 1948 and 1950. Dr. Cannon then entered the private practice of neurological surgery in Memphis, Tennessee. He keenly felt the need of a national neurosurgical society that would admit neurosurgeons soon after completion of their training. He met with several other young neurosurgeons who felt a similar need and he became chairman *pro tem* of the organizing group. He became a founding member of the Congress of Neurological Surgeons (CNS) when this group met in St. Louis on May 10, 1951. Dr. Bland Cannon was the first secretary of the Congress and served as president of the CNS in 1956 at the meeting in Chicago.

Dr. Cannon was certified by the American Board of Neurological Surgery in 1952 and he became a Fellow of the American College of Surgeons in 1953. He became president of the Tennessee Medical Association in 1963 and served in the House of Delegates of the American Medical Association (AMA) from 1965 to 1975. He was a member of the Council on Medical Education of the AMA between 1965 and 1975 and he became special advisor to the chancellor on professional affairs at the University of Tennessee Center of the Health Sciences from 1972 to 1980. He was promoted to clinical professor of neurosurgery at the University of Tennessee. He became chairman of the Department of Neurosurgery at the Baptist Memorial Hospital in Memphis and was vice chancellor for Academic Affairs *pro tem*, of the University of Tennessee Center for Health Sciences in 1974. He was on the Developmental Council of the University of Tennessee between 1975 and 1990. He was on the Medical

Advisory Board of Arthur Young & Company from 1983 to 1986. He became a consultant to the Bureau of Health Insurance of the Social Security Administration and he became a consultant to the Division of Comprehensive Health planning for the Public Health Service.

Dr. Cannon continued in the active practice of neurological surgery until 1980. He then retired to pursue a business career. He is now president of Associated Health Consultants Inc. and is a partner in Cannon, Austin and Cannon, Incorporated, which is a real estate development company. He is a trustee of Rhodes College and is on the Board of Governors of the Institute of Living in Hartford, Connecticut. He is advisor of the Memphis-Shelby County International Airport Authority and is chairman of research and development, Chatanooga Group, Inc.

Dr. Cannon received the Award for Service of the House of Delegates of the AMA in 1973 and the L. M. Graves Health Award in 1973. He received the Mid-South Medical Center Council Award for Leadership and Service and the Certificate of Recognition of the CNS in 1975. He was given a Resolution of Appreciation by the Memphis-Shelby County International Airport Authority in 1978 and received the Bartlett Recognition Award, Foundation for Physical Therapy in 1989. Dr. Cannon has published articles dealing with basic neurophysiological and clinical neurosurgical research. His publications also include philosophical treatises. Dr. Cannon married Louise Shrader Cannon who received her B.A. degree from Carleton College in 1941.

Dr. Cannon has homes in both Memphis, Tennessee and in Florida.

1957

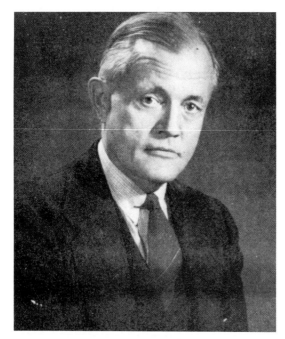

FRANCIS C. GRANT

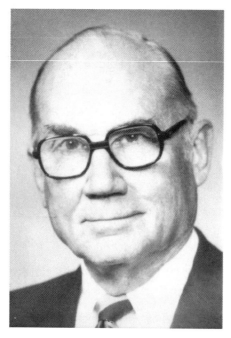

FREDERICK C. REHFELDT

Francis C. Grant

Francis C. Grant, the distinguished guest of honor in 1957, was born in Philadelphia, November 9, 1891. He received an A.B. degree from Harvard University in 1914 and his M.D. degree from the University of Pennsylvania in 1919. He was an intern at the Hospital at the University of Pennsylvania and went on to become a resident in general surgery under Dr. Charles H. Frazier. It was at this time that he received his initial stimulus into neurosurgery. Dr. Frazier was beginning to establish a large neurosurgical service, and Dr. Grant remained in training at the University Hospital and concentrated in this field. He next spent a year with Dr. Cushing in Boston to increase his knowledge of neurosurgical problems. Upon his return to Philadelphia he became chief of neurosurgery at the Graduate Hospital at the University of Pennsylvania where he remained until 1936. On the death of Dr. Frazier, Dr. Grant became professor of neurosurgery at the University of Pennsylvania. Dr. Grant was a skilled operator combining technical ability and great emphasis on postoperative care. He special fields of interest centered around the surgery of brain tumors and of intractable pain. One of his publications on the subject of brain tumors is a review of over 2400 cases which he studied carefully and evaluated from the point of view of morbidity and mortality and their relationship to pathological type.

Dr. Grant always enjoyed teaching undergraduates and residents. In the prior field he placed great emphasis on the development of a seminar-type class in which he did the teaching himself, establishing great rapport with the students. The author of over 200 papers in his specialty, Dr. Grant was considered an outstanding neurosurgeon by his colleagues both here and on the Continent as is well attested by his membership in many honorary neurosurgical societies. Dr. Francis Grant died in November 1967.

GEORGE M. AUSTIN, M.D.

Frederick C. Rehfeldt

Frederick C. Rehfeldt was born in Jackson, Mississippi on July 1, 1915. His father was a physician. He attended the Millsap College between 1932 and 1936. He graduated from the Tulane University School of Medicine in 1941. His house officer training was at the Tulane Unit of Charity Hospital and at the Ochsner Foundation in New Orleans, Louisiana. Dr. Rehfeldt served on active duty in the United States Navy Reserves during World War II and he rose to the rank of lieutenant commander. He became chief of the Division of Neurology and Psychiatry at the United States Navy Mobile Hospital #9 in Oran, Algiers and then became chief of the Division of Neurology and Psychiatry for the Mediterranean Theatre. He received the Secretary of the Navy Commendation for action at Gela and Salerno. He later was transferred to Bethesda National Naval Medical Center in Washington, DC.

Dr. Rehfeldt became a founding member of the Congress of Neurological Surgeons. The founders learned that it was important to prepare a critique of the prior meeting and to prepare an annual meeting manual in great detail. The founders also discovered the importance of audiovisual teams. Dr. Rehfeldt was president of the Congress in 1957, when a very successful meeting was held in Washington, DC.

Dr. Rehfeldt was chief of staff of the Harris Hospital between 1955 and 1960. He was president of the Tulane Medical Alumni in Texas and became director of the Carter Blood Center. He became chairman of the board of the Orme School in Mayer, Arizona and was chairman of the board of Justin Industries. He was elected a member of the Fort Worth City Council and served between 1969 and 1971. He was chairman of the Texas Board of Human Resources. He was a director of the Continental National Bank. He became a charter member of the American Academy of Medical Directors and has been a member of the Southwest Historical Society. He owns, exhibits, and rides quarter horses and collects clipper ship models.

Dr. Rehfeldt married Ethel Evan Bennett on June 24, 1942. The Rehfeldts have a daughter Ethel Rehfeldt DeMarr and a son, Frederick A. Rehfeldt.

1958

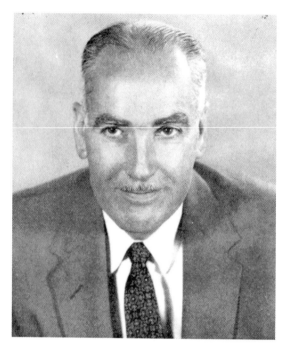

A. Earl Walker

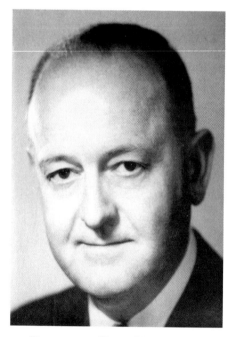

Raymond Kief Thompson

A. Earl Walker

A. Earl Walker, the distinguished guest of honor in 1958, was born in Winnipeg, Canada, in 1907. He graduated from both the undergraduate and medical schools of the University of Alberta.

He interned at the Provincial Mental Institution of Edmonton, Alberta, from 1929 to 1930 and at the Toronto Western Hospital in Toronto, Ontario, Canada, from 1930 to 1931.

As this volume shows, his background in neurologic surgery was firmly established under an outstanding neurologist, Dr. Roy Grinker; a Cushing-trained, original thinking, neurologic surgeon, Dr. Percival Bailey; and one of the fathers of American neurophysiology, Dr. John Fulton, at Yale. He served his residency in neurologic surgery at the University of Chicago Clinics, and from 1935 to 1936 he was a Rockefeller Fellow in Neurophysiologic Research at Yale. He held a position in neuroanatomic research at the Neurologische Klinik in Amsterdam, Holland, in 1937 and in the same year did research in neurophysiology at Brussels, Belgium.

From 1937 to 1947 he was professor of neurosurgery at the University of Chicago and in charge of this section, and in 1947 he was made the neurosurgeon-in-chief at The Johns Hopkins Hospital in Baltimore, Maryland. His predecessors in this particular position included Harvey Cushing and Walter Dandy. During his training period in neurophysiology he published a text, *The Primate Thalamus*, which has been regarded as one of the outstanding contributions about the thalamus.

He has been regarded as both a thinking and practical surgeon of outstanding ability. He has always been a recognized authority on electroencephalography and has been one of the chief contributors in this field in the past. His bibliography at the age of 52 includes several texts and over 200 articles concerning various phases of neurologic surgery. His clinical interest and originality in epilepsy and surgery of the brain stem have taken firm background from experimental work performed in Dr. Fulton's laboratory.

During World War II he was in charge of the Neurosurgical Section of the Cushing General Hospital. All of the cases of posttraumatic epilepsy from the United States Army were sent to this hospital for evaluation. His statistics, which have been published recently, have constituted an extremely informative series of facts about posttraumatic epilepsy with a follow-up period of 10 years.

His resident and laboratory staffs at The Johns Hopkins Hospital have included men from many parts of the world. He has insisted on his men being well grounded in neurologic surgery and all of its allied fields. He has been extremely active in experimental work in the past and has also been extremely active in international neurosurgical circles, being asked to give lectureships on an honorary basis throughout various countries of the globe.

ROBERT G. FISHER, M.D.

Raymond Kief Thompson

Raymond Kief Thompson was born in Vermillion, South Dakota on June 16, 1916, the son of a college professor. His early years were spent in New York City. With his family he moved to Maryland in 1920 and it has been his home ever since. With the untimely death of his father and the Great Depression, education was a cherished ideal obtained only when employment afforded sufficient funds to make further education possible. Medical school had to be interrupted between the sophomore and junior years to earn sufficient funds to complete the training. In 1941 he graduated from the University of Maryland School of Medicine with honors. His house staff training as a rotating intern was followed by being invited to train in neurological surgery with Dr. Charles Bagley, Jr. at the University of Maryland.

Dr. Thompson served as a lieutenant in the United States Naval Reserves during World War II. He ended his Naval career after serving at the National Naval Medical Center in Bethesda, Maryland. After the war he joined the faculty at the University of Maryland and continued to progress up the academic ladder until 1985 when he was awarded the title, Professor Emeritus of Surgery (Neurosurgery).

In 1948, he established the Neurosurgical Research Laboratory at the University of Maryland and still continues scientific investigation in this laboratory.

Dr. Thompson has enjoyed the honor of being chosen president of both the Congress of Neurological Surgeons and the Neurosurgical Society of America. He has been awarded Distinguished Practitioner of Neurological Surgery by the Southern Neurosurgical Society. He also serves as Honorary President of the World Federation of Neurosurgical Societies. He also is a trustee of the Foundation for International Education in Neurological Surgery.

The most memorable event while he served the Congress of Neurological Surgeons was, with the help of Mr. Williams of Williams & Wilkins, the establishment of the yearly volume of *Clinical Neurosurgery*. These volumes over the years have honored many of the great in neurological surgery and have become a choice possession of all members of the Congress of Neurological Surgeons.

His lifetime research work on brain stem distortion continues to be the thrust of his investigations into the workings of the nervous system. He continues to enjoy teaching and helping others with their careers in neurological surgery.

1959

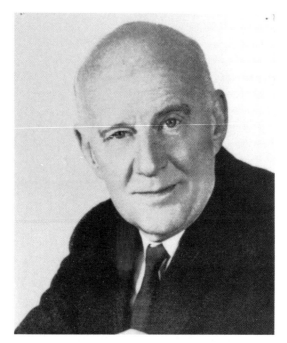

WILLIAM JOHN GERMAN

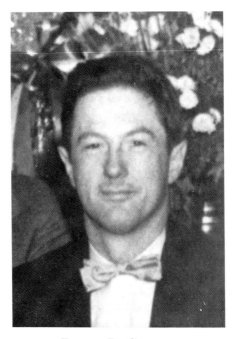

PHILIP D. GORDY

William John German

Our honored guest, Dr. William John German, comes to us as a beloved teacher and respected investigator. His lifetime has been devoted to medicine and to the Cushing tradition in neurosurgery in particular. He was imbued with this spirit through the late Professor S. Harvey, who trained with Dr. Cushing, and later through Dr. Cushing himself when the latter spent his years of retirement at Yale as Sterling Professor of Neurology.

Dr. German was born at McKeesport, Pennsylvania, October 28, 1899. When he was 14 years old his family moved to California, where he received his undergraduate education, earning the A.B. degree at the University of California at Berkeley in 1922. The following year he received his M.A. degree from the same institution, at the same time fulfilling the requirements of the first year of medical school. He then transferred to Harvard, which conferred upon him in 1926 the M.D. degree *magna cum laude.* Yale awarded him an honorary M.A. degree in 1948. While in medical school he belonged to the Alpha Kappa fraternity, and recently he was made an honorary member of the Yale chapter of Alpha Omega Alpha.

His surgical internship was served at the Peter Bent Brigham Hospital from 1926 to 1927, and the following year was spent in Baltimore as a fellow in surgery at The Johns Hopkins Hospital. He served as assistant resident and resident in neurosurgery and surgery under Dr. Harvey at the New Haven Hospital from 1928 to 1931. He was appointed chief of neurosurgery at the New Haven Hospital in 1933. In this capacity he was part of the faculty of the Yale University School of Medicine, serving as instructor from 1930 to 1932; assistant professor from 1932 to 1938, during which time he worked with Harvey Cushing, who had come to Yale in 1934; associate professor from 1938 to 1948; and professor since 1948. His clinical acumen, sound judgment, and appreciation of patients as people have eminently qualified him for the leading position he holds in Connecticut medicine.

During World War II he entered the Navy as a lieutenant commander and shortly thereafter, upon his transfer to Hawaii, was given a spot promotion to commander. He served from 1944 to 1946 but has always managed to maintain his interest in the Navy. He retired in 1959 with the rank of captain, in which capacity he also served as officer-in-charge of the Naval Reserve Medical Company, New Haven, Connecticut. Maintaining the Naval tradition in the family are his oldest son, William, who in 1959 was serving with the rank of ensign on active duty, and his second son, John, who at the same time was a second year medical student at Yale serving in the Medical Reserve.

Dr. German had many affiliations with professional societies, several of which he served in administrative posts. He was president in 1953 of the Harvey Cushing Society, of which he was a charter member; vice president of the Society of Neurological Surgeons in 1955; and secretary-treasurer of the American Board of Neurological Surgeons from 1947 to 1952. In addition, he was a member of the American Medical Association, American Neurological Association, New England Neurosurgical Society, Society of University Surgeons, and Association for Research in Nervous and Mental Diseases.

Bacon declared that "men should enter upon learning in order to give a true account of their gift of reason to the benefit and use of men." Through his influence upon a generation of medical students and a host of graduate students extending in numbers far beyond his own residents, Dr. German fulfilled the destiny of his gift and has attained a unique position as an outstanding teacher of neurosurgery.

His method of teaching was characterized largely by a system of guidance for a man's own intellectual growth. No man has been forced into a mold. In this respect he was akin to Socrates, who compared his own method to midwifery, for as it is the mother who labors and gives birth, so it is the student who is primarily active in the process of learning. The teacher merely assists in a natural process which might otherwise be more painful and might possibly fail without such help. This teaching takes place in an unhurried atmosphere, for Dr. German realized early in his career that no man could do everything. Therefore it was necessary to recognize what had to be done and to do that much well. Yet he always had time for the problems, both professional and personal, of his residents. Both he and Mrs. German welcomed at all times each resident into their home. Thus, those residents who served under Dr. German always felt a close and warm relationship with their chief.

His standing as a teacher stemmed, perhaps, from his never having ceased to be himself a student. He was always willing to accept new ideas and techniques, but in accepting them he tempered them with patience, judgment, and keen evaluation of their merit by an incisive insight into the core of the problem unfettered by nonessential facts. The breadth and scope of his interests are apparent in his bibliography. Quality rather than galley proof mileage were his aim, and he often advised ambitious authors to file their articles in the bottom drawer for a year, at the end of which time, if the paper still read well, it would be fit for publication and none the worse for the delay.

As a practitioner he showed a deep understanding of human nature and never allowed the neurosurgical problem to overshadow the patient's importance as a whole person. The little comforts so significant to the sick did not escape his notice, and he showed patient respect for the personal dignity of those entrusted to his care. I have drawn a picture of an outstanding person, in some ways perhaps a saint, but his attitude was so self-effacing that the patient always remained the primary figure. This quality is best exemplified in the story of one resident who mentioned at a conference that he had operated upon the patient. He was told later that at this institution we say the patient was operated upon. Dr. William German died in January 1981.

LYCURGUS M. DAVEY, M.D.

Philip D. Gordy

Dr. Gordy received his M.D. from the University of Michigan Medical School in 1943. Following this he served an internship and assistant residency in surgery at The New York Hospital. During this period he came under the influence of Dr. Bronson Ray. Upon completion of this service, he entered the

Army Medical Corps and, after the usual initial period of training, he was sent overseas where he served in France and Germany. Though his service at Cornell had been in general surgery, every overseas assignment placed him on another neurosurgical service. First he was assigned to the neurosurgical service in Paris under Dr. Edgar A. Kahn. After several months there he was reassigned to Frankfurt, Germany where he served under Dr. Sid Gross from Mt. Sinai in New York. After transfer back to France, where he served as Chief of Surgery of the 78th Field Hospital, he was active in both general and neurosurgery.

After discharge from the Army in 1946, Dr. Gordy returned to his hometown of Ann Arbor where he was accepted as a resident in neurosurgery. His mentors at Ann Arbor were Dr. Max Peet, Dr. Edgar Kahn, and Dr. Robert Bassett. The many distinguished neurosurgical visitors to the service at Michigan were also a significant influence on his neurosurgical development. His neurosurgical training was completed in 1949. During the training period he obtained a Master's degree in neuroanatomy under Dr. Elizabeth Crosby.

After searching about for a suitable place in which to establish a practice, he visited Wilmington, Delaware; this appeared to be the ideal place, despite the fact that it was only 25 miles from Philadelphia, one of the strongholds of neurosurgery. Doctors Grant, Groff, and Scott all proved to be of great help and support to the young whippersnapper who had invaded their territory. A strong and busy practice was developed and Dr. Gordy was eventually joined, first by Dr. Livio Olmedo and then by Dr. Ray Hillyard.

Close ties were maintained with the services in Philadelphia. Dr. Gordy and his associate, Dr. Olmedo, were deeply involved in the training of the general surgical residents as they rotated through the neurosurgical service. A significant number of the residents made the decision to enter the field of neurosurgery as a result of the dedication to teaching that they encountered on the service. Doctors Gordy and Olmedo were, on more than one occasion, and in a good-humored vein, accused of stealing all the surgical residents!

In an effort to keep abreast of rapidly developing developments in the field, Dr. Gordy attended as many meetings as possible. This led to a wide acquaintance with other young neurosurgeons around the country and, eventually, to becoming a member of the group that met in St. Louis in 1951 to form the Congress of Neurological Surgeons.

Dr. Gordy was one of the founding members of the Congress of Neurological Surgeons in 1951. Active participation in the affairs of the Congress, through committee assignments, led eventually to membership on the executive committee and then to the positions of secretary-treasurer, vice president and then, in 1959, to the position of president.

The choice of a meeting site for 1959 was Miami Beach, Florida. The honored guest for this meeting was Dr. William J. German, professor of neurosurgery at Yale University. Dr. German was a unique individual and a delight to all who knew him. His manner of teaching his residents was one of gentleness and example, always stressing the need to look for the scientific basis of disease conditions. Sound clinical judgment, a keen insight into problems of the nervous system, and an appreciation of the patient as a person were hallmarks of his approach to neurosurgery.

The major theme of the Miami Beach meeting was related to the various aspects of brain tumors. The officers and members of the Congress found it a stimulating meeting and Dr. German lived up to his well-deserved reputation as a teacher of neurosurgery.

At the time of this meeting Dr. Gordy had been in practice in Wilmington, Delaware since 1949. By 1963 he felt a growing urge to leave the field of private practice and enter academic neurosurgery. Having had the opportunity to teach residents who rotated onto neurosurgery from general surgery in Wilmington, the next step seemed to be obtaining an academic position from which his interest in teaching could be more effective. The opportunity came with an appointment as associate professor of neurosurgery at The University of Oregon. Dr. George Austin was chairman of the department. Promotion to full professor occurred in due time.

After 3 years at Oregon, Dr. Gordy was requested to assume the position of Chairman of the Division of Neurosurgery at Thomas Jefferson University Hospital in Philadelphia. During his tenure at Jefferson, Dr. Gordy restructured neurosurgery as a separate department. His service at that institution was noted for solid teaching in clinical neurosurgery, patient care, operative techniques, and for the development of city-wide neurosurgical conferences.

An auxiliary service was developed in Wilmington, Delaware through which the residents rotated to amplify their clinical operative experience. This service was directed locally by Dr. Gordy's former associate, Dr. Livio Olmedo, who was a superb technical neurosurgeon and a gifted teacher. The Jefferson service was approved by the American Board of Neurosurgery for two residents each year. A large number of residents were graduated from the service and are now practicing in various areas of the country.

After 7 years at Jefferson, Dr. Gordy made the difficult decision to leave Jefferson and return to private practice. This was occasioned largely for health reasons, but also by reason of a desire to return to the West and to resume private practice. Casper, Wyoming was suggested by some neurosurgical colleagues who recognized the town's need for a competent neurosurgeon. The move was made in January 1973, just in time for one of the worst snowstorms the area had experienced in many years, and which has not been equaled since! Casper proved to be an excellent medical community and Dr. Gordy developed a busy and well-recognized service. He was later joined by one of his former residents from the Jefferson service.

His wife, Silvia, opened The Oregon Trail Fine Arts Gallery which became a well-recognized gallery throughout the West. The gallery adjoined Dr. Gordy's office and afforded patients a variation on the usual waiting room tedium by giving them the opportunity to wander through the various gallery rooms and to enjoy the paintings and sculptures that were on display. When not in the operating room, making rounds, or in the office, Dr. Gordy was frequently called upon to do the crating and shipping for the gallery!

Dr. Gordy made the difficult decision to retire from active neurosurgery in 1984. In this same year, he recognized the need for a rehabilitation service in Casper, and proposed to the hospital board that such a service be developed. The proposal was accepted, and Dr. Gordy served a "mini-residency" in Rehabilitation Medicine at St. Joseph's Hospital in Albuquerque. He then served as medical director of the service until 1986 at which time he retired once again! His colleagues in the operating room and on the rehabilitation service commented that he retired so often because he liked the retirement parties so much! In fact he was given a plaque on which were fastened crossed Adson elevators with the caption below saying, *"Never again!"*

Since 1986 Dr. Gordy has been busy with writing, woodworking, dubbing around on the violin and the viola, and periodic participation in medicolegal defense work. He and Silvia enjoy traveling, especially in the Rocky Mountains and in Spain (when the retirement funds permit). They are also amateur archeologists and pursue that interest whenever Wyoming weather permits. Silvia continues to sell some art from their extensive collection, left over from when the gallery was closed. It seems only yesterday that the 11 "young turks" assembled in St. Louis and proposed the revolutionary idea of a new neurosurgical society devoted primarily to the special interests and needs of "the younger neurosurgeon." Dr. Gordy seriously doubts that we can continue to think of ourselves in that category. However, to see what has developed, with the status of the Congress of Neurological Surgeons as one of the great neurosurgical organizations of the world; its close cooperation with the American Association of Neurological Surgeons; and its emphasis on neurosurgical excellence in teaching, research, and socio-economic development for the betterment of the neurosurgical patients; makes him proud indeed to be a part of the 40th anniversary celebration of the Congress of Neurological Surgeons.

1960

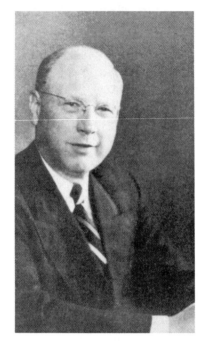

PAUL C. BUCY

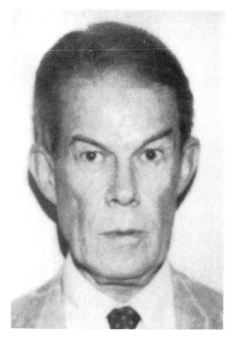

THOMAS M. MARSHALL

Paul C. Bucy

Dr. Paul C. Bucy, the honored guest of the 1960 meeting of the Congress of Neurological Surgeons, is a long-time friend of this organization. Dr. Bucy generously served as a principal speaker at the first (and the only unpublished) meeting of the Congress in 1951.

Born in Hubbard, Iowa, on November 13, 1904, Dr. Bucy wasted no time in pursuing the studies which led to his attainment of eminence in the neurological world. By his 23rd birthday he had: earned his B.S. and M.D. degrees and the degree of M.S. in neuropathology at the State University of Iowa; seen his first scientific publication in print; and started internship at the Henry Ford Hospital in Detroit. He had also courted and married his wife, Evelyn. The two had met over the telephone wires when they were both rural exchange operators.

In 1928, Dr. Bucy joined Dr. Percival Bailey's newly created neurosurgical staff at the University of Chicago, as its first resident, becoming an instructor two years later. In 1930 and 1931, as a traveling fellow, he worked under Dr. Gordon Holmes at the National Hospital, Queen Square, London, and under Dr. Otfrid Foerster in Breslau, Germany. In 1933 he carried out an extensive program of neurophysiological research in the laboratory of the late Dr. John F. Fulton at Yale University. Upon returning to the University of Chicago, Dr. Bucy remained on the neurosurgical staff, rising to rank of associate professor, being in charge of neurological surgery beginning in 1939.

In 1941 Dr. Bucy left the University of Chicago and entered private practice, working at Chicago Memorial Hospital, where he was chief of staff for 11 years. In 1954 he began his clinical practice at Chicago Wesley Memorial Hospital, where he is in charge of the division of neurological surgery. However, he has continued to be most active as a teacher, being professor of neurology and neurological surgery at the University of Illinois until 1954 and since then professor of surgery at Northwestern University. Although he is expert and fluent as a didactic lecturer, Dr. Bucy's teaching of his residents stresses careful and thorough observation of patients. His intense interest in clinical neurosurgical problems stimulates in his residents a thirst for more and more understanding in this field.

The diversity of Dr. Bucy's neurological interests is proved by the wide variety of subjects dealt with in his bibliography. He has made important contributions to knowledge in the fields of neuropathology, neurophysiology, clinical neurology, and neurological surgery. He has participated in the writing of the classic volumes, *Intracranial Tumors of Infancy and Childhood* (with Percival Bailey and Douglas Buchanan), *The Precentral Motor Cortex*, and *Neurology* (with Roy Grinker and Adolph Sahs). A member of the Literary Club of Chicago, Dr. Bucy has also written fascinating accounts of some of the colorful characters of early midwestern America overlooked by other historians.

Dr. Bucy has long been a leader in neurology and neurological surgery. He helped found the Harvey Cushing Society, was elected as its president in 1951, and is presently its director of publications. He has been chairman of the Section on Nervous and Mental Diseases of the American Medical Association, president of the Chicago Neurological Society, and vice president of the Chicago Surgical Society. He was made vice president of the American Neurological Association in 1954. From 1943 to 1947 he served as secretary-treasurer of the American Board of Neurological Surgery.

In recent years Dr. Bucy has been concerned with the development of neurological surgery abroad. He has made extensive trips, visiting neurological surgeons in Europe, the Near East, the Far East, and South America. He participated in the formation of the World Federation of Neurosurgical Societies and has served as its president (1957–1961).

As a man of scientific distinction, a master surgeon with vast clinical experience, a great teacher, a leader of neurological surgeons. Dr. Bucy could well be respected for these traits alone. But his pupils, patients, and colleagues will testify to his kindness, his utter lack of affectation, and his forthright honesty, which engender confidence and endear him to all.

JOHN R. RUSSELL, M.D.

Thomas M. Marshall

Thomas M. Marshall was born in 1917 to Mr. and Mrs. Wiley Marshall in Frankfort, Kentucky where his father was an attorney. During early school years, an interest in music was pursued on the French horn and by playing trumpet in several dance bands. After receiving an A.B. degree from the University of Kentucky, where the horn and trumpet playing continued, he entered the University of Louisville School of Medicine. Between the sophomore and junior years, he formed a band with four fellow medical students and played abroad ships to Europe. He was elected to Alpha Omega Alpha and received an M.D. degree in 1941.

During internship at Louisville General Hospital, Dr. Marshall courted and married Nancye Miller, a nursing supervisor at Children's Hospital. Two weeks later he was on sea duty with the United States Navy. After this tour of duty, a six-month crash course at St. Elizabeth's Hospital in Washington, D.C. followed, and he practiced psychiatry until released from the Navy in 1946. After returning to Louisville General Hospital for some general surgery training, Dr. Marshall received neurosurgical training at the Mayo Clinic and was awarded an M.S. degree in neurosurgery from the University of Minnesota and was elected to the Society of Sigma Xi.

Dr. Marshall returned to Louisville and was associated with Dr. Franklin Jelsma for 3 years before entering solo practice. Shortly thereafter, he was a founding member of the Congress of Neurological Surgeons and was its president in 1960. The annual meeting of the Congress at Chicago with Dr. Paul Bucy as the honored guest, was the highlight of the year. In addition to private practice, he was an associate clinical professor of neurological surgery at the University of Louisville School of Medicine. He has served as president of the medical staff of several Louisville hospitals and continues to be active in civic organizations. After retirement from the active practice of neurosurgery in 1988, he has continued his interest in neurosurgery as a consultant in disability evaluations. Retirement has afforded opportunities to pursue the hobbies of tennis, fishing, and traveling.

He and Nancye have raised two girls and a boy, and now proudly exclaim the virtues of a grandson.

1961

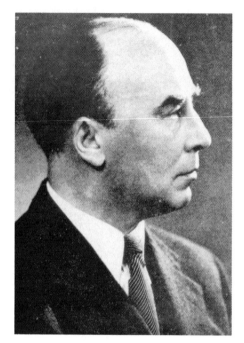

Eduard A. V. Busch

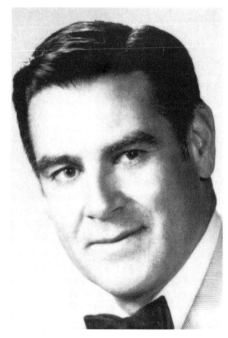

Martin Peter Sayers

Eduard A. V. Busch

When it was decided to invite Dr. Eduard Busch as our honored guest for the meeting in New York in 1961, a man was chosen who was rather accustomed to receiving high professional honors.

He was an honorary member of: The British Society of Neurological Surgeons; La Societé de Neurochirurgie de Langue Française; Sociedad Chilena de Neurologia, Psiquitria y Neurocirurgia; Sociedad de Cirurjanos de Hospital Chile; Sociedad Medica de Santiago; Sociedad de Neuropsiquitria y Medicina Legal de Valparaiso; Associacion Medica Argentina; III° Congresso Sul-Americano de Neuro-Cirurgia; IV° Congresso Sul-Americano de Neuro-Cirurgia, Tokyo Bay Medical Society; Societa Italiana de Neuro-Chirurgia; Societé de Chirurgie de Lyon; Asamblea Nacional de Cirurjanos; y Conferencia Mexicana de Neurologia Quirurgia. He also is an honorary professor of the Facultad de Biologia y Ciensias Medicas de la Universidad de Chile. Furthermore, Dr. Busch was made an Honorary Consultant of Neurosurgery at the 3rd, 5th, and 15th ROK Army Hospitals, of Korea Police Hospital, of POW Hospital, Pusan, and of the Children's Hospital, Pusan. He was awarded the American Medal of Freedom 3, United Nations Medal of Honor, Storkors af den Islandske Falk (Iceland) and Storkors af den Islandske Falk med Stjerne (Iceland), Ridder af Danebrog (Denmark), Ridder af 1.grad af Danebrog (Denmark), Jutlandia Medaljen (Denmark) and Dansk Kirurgisk Selskabs Mindemedalje (Denmark), and finally he was awarded two great Danish honorary grants. To make the record complete it should be mentioned that Dr. Busch on his way from Denmark to our meeting in New York had to make a stopover in Iceland to be made an Honorary Doctor of Medicine at the University of Iceland.

In spite of all previous honors bestowed upon him Dr. Busch was particularly pleased to accept the invitation as the honored guest of the Congress of Neurological Surgeons, and he was so, for two reasons: First, because he was always a great admirer of North America, its people, and its traditions. Many of his closest friends were Americans, and to him as to all other neurosurgeons this is the place where the cradle of neurosurgery stood. This is the land of Drs. Cushing, Dandy, Frazier, Mixter, Naffziger, Horrax, Peet, Adson, and others whose names forever will be remembered among neurosurgeons. It is also the land that still possesses so many outstanding men in the field of neurosurgery and allied sciences, toward whom most of the neurosurgical attention of the world is directed. It is, therefore, rightfully considered a great honor for a man from abroad to be invited as the guest of honor of one of the outstanding neurosurgical societies of this country.

The second reason for Dr. Busch to feel pleased by receiving an invitation from the Congress of Neurological Surgeons was because the unique type of meetings conducted by this society appealed to him—the type of meeting in which the emphasis is placed upon passing to the younger neurosurgeons the experiences of the older ones, the meetings planned to bridge the past with the future in the field of neurological surgery. Dr. Busch always considered teaching as one of the main objects of the pioneers of neurosurgery.

Dr. Busch was born in Copenhagen, Denmark, on September 9, 1899—an unusual birthday for an unusual man. Once he was asked by a police officer in London to give his name and birthday. When the officer heard the date 9/9/99, he asked sarcastically: "Did you give a wrong name, too?" Dr. Busch did his undergraduate work and went to medical school in Copenhagen where he received his M.D. degree in 1924 from the University of Copenhagen. In 1930 his dissertation, "Studies on the Nerves of the Blood-Vessels, with Especial Reference to Periarterial Sympathectomy," was accepted by the University of Copenhagen, and he was made Doctor of Medicinae. After medical school he went into general surgery, in which field he received excellent training from three outstanding Danish general surgeons: Johannes Ipsen, Mogens Fenger, and Vilhelm Schaldemose. Following his training in general surgery he was licensed by the Board of General Surgery in 1932. During his training in general surgery he played with the idea of going into neurosurgery but discarded the idea again because he felt that from a therapeutic standpoint neurological surgery was a rather hopeless field! During the later part of his training in general surgery, however, he had the opportunity to operate upon a boy with a cranial-cerebral injury. Finding how remarkably well the boy made out he changed his attitude, and encouraged by Schaldemose, who pointed out to him the great demand for surgeons specialized in this field, he decided to go into neurosurgery. It was planned that he should take his neurosurgical training in Paris with Petit-Dutaillis. Before doing so he went on a vacation to Sweden, where he stopped in to see Dr. Olivecrona in Stockholm. Dr. Busch became so impressed by the work done by Olivecrona that he decided to take his training there. He spent 1½ years with Olivecrona learning Olivecrona's excellent clinical and surgical methods. The stay there resulted in a very close friendship between these two men which lasted ever since.

Following his stay in Stockholm Dr. Busch went on a trip to the United States, where he studied neurological surgery for 3 months. He went to see Dr. Cushing and followed the work being done on Dr. Cushing's service. He was appointed Dr. Cushing's professional "nephew." Dr. Busch also visited Dr. Dandy and was invited to stay in Dandy's home as a house guest. The meeting with these two outstanding neurological surgeons made a great impression on the young visitor, and he considered it one of his greatest experiences.

Upon his return to Denmark he was made a staff member in neurology at the University Hospital in Copenhagen, because neurosurgery was not considered important enough to be made a speciality of its own; and, of course, the idea was that the diagnosis should be made by a neurologist anyhow! Dr. Busch was given 11 beds from the professor of neurology, Viggo Christiansen. He got one assistant and his monthly salary was $70.00, which was considered plenty for the two or three neurosurgical patients he was expected to be treating per month. Of course, once the neurosurgeon was available the demand for neurosurgical treatment increased rapidly. In 1939 he was made head of his own service at the University Hospital, but not until 1948 was neurological surgery given its own professorship in Denmark and Dr. Busch was made the first professor in this field. His service now has about 80 beds, there are a dozen doctors working there, and through the years Dr. Busch's service has treated 30,000 to 40,000 neurosurgical patients. Dr. Busch was very active in establishing other neurosurgical services in Denmark, and in 1961 Denmark had six such services, all headed by men who trained with Dr. Busch.

During the war Dr. Busch was active in the underground movement against the German occupation; he was probably inspired by one of his very close friends, the professor of neurology, Dr. Mogens Fog, who was one of the top leaders of the underground movement. During the Korean War Dr. Busch was among those who organized the Danish hospital ship, Jutlandia, which was sent to Korea as part of the Danish help to the United Nations. Dr. Busch went with the ship as head of the neurosurgical service. During his stay in Korea he not only did a great amount of work on the ship but he also organized neurosurgical services ashore for both the armed forces and the Korean people. He took a special interest in the Children's Hospital. In this work he received help from a neurosurgical friend in the United States to whom he wrote: "You are working in one of the best equipped hospitals in the world. I am working in one of the poorest. I need your help"—and he received plenty.

Dr. Busch was a founding member of the Scandinavian Society of Neurosurgery and he was the first vice president of the Society and the second president. He was a member of Dansk Oto-Neuro-Ofthalmologisk Selskab, Dansk Neurologisk Selskab, Dansk Medicinsk Selskab, Deutsches Gesellschaft für Chirurgie, Svensk Neurologisk Forening, Det Islandske Videnskabernes Selskab, and a corresponding member of the Harvey Cushing Society. He was president for the Third International Congress of Neurological Surgery held in Copenhagen in 1965.

Dr. Busch had a very dynamic personality. He was a very charming person, but may have also caused controversy mainly because of his dynamic approach to problems. He thought fast and acted fast, and he expected others to do the same. He was not an ordinary type of person and he always made a strong impression on those who met him and especially on those who got to know him closely. He was a strong believer in the democratic principles, in political life as well as in his own department. It was apparent to those working with him, however, that for a chief with such a powerful personality it frequently was difficult to transfer theoretical ideas about democracy into practical life in the department. He required hard and long working hours from his associates and if the work was not done to his satisfaction he would let them know so. To those who worked with him he remained a close friend, and he always took a keen interest in the future of his associates. Nobody ever asked for his help or advice in vain. First of all he was a very warmhearted man, devoted to his work, his patients, his family, and his friends. He sincerely disliked personal glorifying, and the writer took a great personal risk of attracting his dislike by listing all his honorary degrees and especially by mentioning them at the beginning of this biography.

Dr. Busch was devoted to his patients. He wanted them treated on a very personal level—more like close friends than like patients in a big hospital. He liked to compare his service with that of the country doctor, who knew not only the medical problems of the patient but also his whole personal background. His interest for the patient extended to the relatives of the patient too. He always emphasized the impact of a serious disease on the patient and his relatives and the fact that the problem should be dealt with accordingly. Although he made rounds fast he always had a kind remark for each patient. Dr. Busch was a gifted surgeon and, although his motto was "An operation is soon enough done when good enough done," his surgical procedures were done fast as everything else he did.

Among the many associates Dr. Busch had through the years were also many from abroad who came to spend shorter or longer periods of time with him and who, when they left, took with them something, but who also left their marks on the department.

Dr. Busch's main hobbies apart from his professional work (which did not leave him too much time for other hobbies) were golf and deer hunting. He was a personal friend of the Danish king and he frequently participated in the royal hunts.

In 1937 he married Rigmor Schaeffer, an unusually fine lady, known for her kindness and hospitality. She was the gracious hostess for their many friends, professional and personal—be they from Denmark or from abroad—gathering in their delightful home. Dr. and Mrs. Busch raised two attractive children, a daughter, Hanne, and a son, Aksel.

Mrs. Busch was a trained physical therapist and, before she married the doctor, spent 7 years in the United States. During her stay in the States she was the personal physical therapist to Franklin D. Roosevelt after he contracted polio and before he became President of the United States.

I have wanted to draw a picture of a strong and very unusual personality, a man who has left his mark on neurosurgery and on those who have met him. I am not fortunate enough to be able to say that I knew Cushing, but I am proud that I can say, "I knew Busch." Dr. Eduard Busch died in 1982.

PALLE TAARNHØJ, M.D.

Martin Peter Sayers

A Middle Westerner and a graduate of The Ohio State University, Dr. Sayers became, before entering medical school, a close friend of Harry E. LeFever, professor of neurosurgery at the Ohio State University. Through Dr. LeFever's influence he chose Philadelphia General Hospital and the Hospital of the University of Pennsylvania for postgraduate training.

In 1950, Jim Gay, visiting in Philadelphia, extended an invitation for Dr. Sayers to become a Congress of Neurological Surgeons founder. Doctor Sayers was in his last year of training.

Dr. Sayers became the 11th president of the Congress in 1961. This period was one of rapid growth in membership and intensive effort to help young neurosurgeons to become Board certified and to set up a habit of continuing education. The members weeded out a few impostors, forged stronger relationships, and planned joint ventures with the other American neurosurgical societies. The Congress of Neurological Surgeons had become the largest neurosurgical organization in the world at that time.

Dr. Sayers was a pioneer pediatric neurological surgeon. He became assistant professor of neurological surgery at Ohio State in 1953 and chief of pediatric neurosurgery in 1954, establishing one of the country's earliest pediatric neurological surgery services at Columbus Children's Hospital. He was instrumental in starting there, in 1959, the first multidisciplinary central nervous system birth defects clinic in the United States. He helped to establish the Pediatric Section of the American Association of Neurological Surgeons and became the chairman; later he was president of the Neurosurgical Society of America. Academically, he progressed to clinical professor in 1973.

As a young pediatric neurological surgeon, Dr. Sayers helped to push the treatment of myelomeningocele forward to the immediate postnatal period and to improve shunting procedures for hydrocephalus. A number of new and improved procedures were developed and over 30 young neurosurgeons received pediatric training under his supervision.

Pete has two sons, a physician and an airline pilot; two lovely daughters, both attorneys; and 11 grandchildren. He and Marjorie are both quite healthy at this reporting. Since retirement in January 1986, he has been clinical professor emeritus of neurological surgery at The Ohio State University. He gave the third annual Donald D. Matson memorial address, titled "The Limbus of Evolution," at the American Association of Neurological Surgeons meeting in 1989, after retirement.

1962

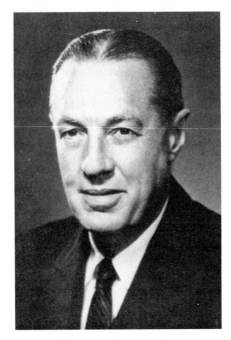

BRONSON SANDS RAY

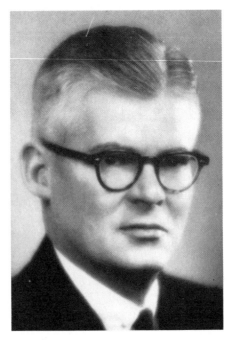

RICHARD L. DeSAUSSURE

Bronson Sands Ray

Our honored guest in 1962, Dr. Bronson Sands Ray, clinical professor of surgery (neurosurgery), Cornell University Medical College, and chief, Department of Neurological Surgery, The New York Hospital, was born January 4, 1904, in New Albany, Indiana. Shortly thereafter his family moved to Fort Wayne, Indiana, where he grew up and attended elementary and secondary schools. He was graduated from Franklin College, Franklin, Indiana, in 1924, *cum laude*, with honors in chemistry. His alma mater in 1950 bestowed upon him the honorary degree of Doctor of Science.

His medical aspirations took him to Northwestern University where he received his M.D. degree in 1928. An early interest in both organic neurology and surgery was kindled perhaps by a brush with poliomyelitis at a young age and by living the formative years in the environment of an active general surgeon, his father, who only at the age of 87 years finally gave up the active practice of medicine in 1961. This interest was undoubtedly further abetted by extra work n neuroanatomy under Dr. Loyal Davis while Dr. Ray was still a medical school freshman, and by additional endeavors as a student assistant in Dr. Stephen W. Ranson's neurophysiological laboratories.

Still undecided as to the exact form his medical career should take, Dr. Ray served a general internship at the Wesley Memorial Hospital and a year as an assistant resident in internal medicine at the Passavant Memorial Hospital, both in Chicago. With the encouragement of Dr. Loyal Davis, he moved on to Boston as surgical house officer at the Peter Bent Brigham Hospital during 1930 and 1931. In 1931 to 1932 he served as Dr. Harvey Cushing's last resident at the Brigham.

Dr. Ray was not convinced that he cared to turn his back on the broader field of surgery and, at the end of his service with Dr. Cushing, went to the newly opened New York Hospital-Cornell University Medical Center in New York, New York. Here he served for the next 4 years, in turn, as assistant resident and resident on the surgical services of the late Dr. George J. Heuer, who in the tradition of his mentor, Dr. William S. Halsted, ran a department of surgery where all phases of surgery were practiced without subdivision. However, soon after Dr. Ray's appointment as attending surgeon to the New York Hospital in 1936, the natural affinity between him and the neurosurgical problems gradually found him, by circumstances if not by design, doing more and more neurological surgery and less and less general surgery as the former made increasing demands on his time. It was not until the mid-1940s, however, that he devoted his efforts completely to neurological surgery.

That this background has served him well is attested by his eminent position in the specialty today. It has undoubtedly convinced him that a solid background in general surgery is a prerequisite to competence in neurological surgery and undoubtedly has molded a career known for its technical excellence and masterful ability to glean from clinical practice knowledge not only regarding individual or series case studies but even basic physiological data, some previously unknown and some formerly erroneously interpreted. During his tenure as chief of the Department of Neurological Surgery at New York Hospital-Cornell University Medical Center he helped to achieve the happy situation of intimate and congenial relationships between neurosurgery and organic neurology. This not always easy conviviality has yielded such basic knowledge as the sources of intracranial pain, and the combined conferences of staff members in these two departments have been both a stimulus and a pleasure to countless medical students and physicians not primarily oriented toward the neurological specialties. Without impinging disproportionately upon the medical school's curriculum, Dr. Ray has by his lectures and conferences provided medical students with a knowledge and, more important, an approach to neurological problems in a form eagerly grasped.

Dr. Ray is now witnessing the fruition of his well conceived career, as evidenced by the innumerable honors and offices he now holds or has held in the recent past, including: secretary-general, Second International Congress of Neurological Surgery; president, Harvey Cushing Society; vice president, American Neurological Association; secretary-treasurer, Society of Neurological Surgeons; representative of the American Neurological Association on the American Board of Neurological Surgery; member, National Research Council, Division of Medical Sciences (Subcommittee on Neurosurgery); delegate from the Society of Neurological Surgery to the World Federation of Neurosurgical Societies; chairman, International Affairs Committee of the World Federation of Neurosurgical Societies; member, Visiting Committee for Department of Medicine, Brookhaven National Laboratory; member, Editorial Board, *Journal of Neurosurgery*; consulting editor as representative in neurosurgery and member of the Advisory Board, *International Abstracts of Surgery, Gynecology and Obstetrics*; and member of the Advisory Council, Neurological Surgeons, American College of Surgeons.

He has impressed upon his residents that their first duty is to their patients, and that, from those committed to their care, they should glean by observation and careful, long-term follow-up whatever the problems present in the way of statistical data as well as basic understanding of disease or physiological processes. He has no quarrel with those who believe that a residency should have a period of laboratory investigation, but he feels that not all are suited to best utilize such time and that risks are inherent in not getting on with the fundamental job of acquiring clinical judgment and technical skill. He has inspired in his residents some of the attitude of the skeptic, taken in its finest sense, to set out to prove no preconceived hypothesis but to evaluate results objectively and to question established opinions if personal observation does not bear out conclusions previously reached by others.

These are but a few of the accomplishments and qualities of this surgeon *par excellence*, objective observer, and commanding personality whose impressions are left indelibly on all those privileged to have had close contact with him.

ROBERT A. CLARK, JR., M.D.

Richard L. DeSaussure, Jr.

Born on the 29th of December 1917 in Macon, Georgia, Dr. DeSaussure's family soon moved to Washington, DC where he graduated from Western High School. He entered the University of Virginia and received an A.B. degree in 1939 and his M.D. degree in 1942. He had a surgical internship at the University of Virginia Hospital and then spent 3 years in the Armed Forces. He was at a Station Hospital in England and later served as a battalion surgeon with the Third Armored Division in France and Germany. Dr. DeSaussure was promoted to major and was awarded the Bronze Star.

Dr. DeSaussure returned to the University of Virginia Hospital where he completed a neurosurgical residency under Dr. Gayle Crutchfield. Next he spent 9 months under Dr. Joseph P. Evans in Cincinnati studying neuropathology and neurophysiology. During this time he met the lovely Phyllis Falk of Washington, DC and married her in July 1948 in the Washington Cathedral. The DeSaussures have three married children and three grandsons. Dr. DeSaussure moved to Memphis in 1949. He was first assistant chief and later chief of neurosurgery at the Kennedy Veterans Hospital. In 1950 Dr. DeSaussure was invited to join Dr. R. Eustace Semmes and Dr. Francis Murphey.

May 1951 was a very important date. Dr. DeSaussure passed the examination of the American Board of Neurological Surgery and in May was asked to join with 21 other neurosurgeons to form the Congress of Neurological Surgeons. Dr. DeSaussure has served as president of the staff of the Baptist Memorial Hospital, vice president of the Memphis & Shelby County Medical Society, speaker of the House of Delegates of the Tennessee Medical Society, chairman of the Advisory Committee for Neurosurgery of the American College of Surgeons, and vice president of the Southern Neurosurgical Society. Dr. DeSaussure became chairman of the Semmes-Murphey Clinic when Dr. Murphey retired. He was appointed medical director of Graduate Medical Education for the Baptist Memorial Hospital during this time. Because of a close affiliation with the University of Tennessee Medical Units he was appointed assistant dean for graduate medical affairs. He has written several papers, the most important of which is "Vascular Injury Co-Incident to Lumbar Disk Surgery."

Dr. DeSaussure was a founding member and for 13 years president of the Mid-South Foundation for Medical Care (the PRO for the State of Tennessee). He has been president of the Memphis Chapter of the English-Speaking Union. He received the "Neurosurgeon Award" from the American Academy of Neurological Surgery in 1972. He received the Award of Appreciation from the University of Tennessee Dental Department and the Dental Society. In 1990 he was honored by being selected a Distinguished Southern Neurosurgeon by the Southern Neurosurgical Society.

Dr. DeSaussure was made an emeritus professor of neurosurgery, University of Tennessee, after retiring from the practice of neurosurgery. However, during this time he served as medical director for a local PPO, Baptist Health Services Group. Dr. DeSaussure retired from all medical activities in March 1991.

1963

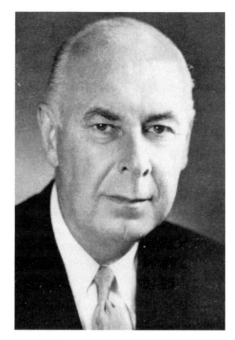

JAMES L. POPPEN

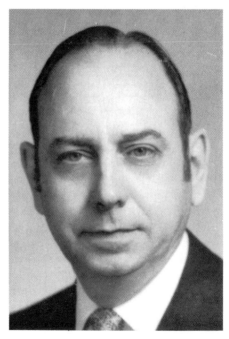

AUSTIN ROY TYRER, JR.

James L. Poppen

James L. Poppen embarked upon his neurosurgical career in 1933 when he joined the staff of the Lahey Clinic. By the time he had completed a 2-year surgical residency at the Illinois Research and Educational Hospital, his major interest seemed to be in neurological surgery although he also trained in general, thoracic, and genitourinary surgery. His formal tutelage in this field, brief by present standards, was provided by Dr. Eric Oldberg.

In the early 1930s the newly formed Lahey Clinic was beginning to expand its surgical and medical practice, and Dr. Frank Lahey quickly recruited Gilbert Horrax to head his neurosurgical department upon Dr. Cushing's retirement from the Peter Bent Brigham Hospital. The long and fruitful association of Drs. Horrax and Poppen is well known and led Dr. Lahey to comment 20 years later, "They have always complemented each other."

But Dr. Poppen's early experiences were disappointing. As a restless and imaginative young surgeon, he was dissatisfied with the tedious and often unrewarding procedures. In addition he deplored the frequent recourse to temporal decompression as a means of dealing with deep-seated brain tumors. His extraordinary skill might have been lost to neurosurgery had it not been for several visits to the clinics of Drs. Dandy, Peet, and Adson where he learned that seemingly inoperable tumors could be removed successfully. He credits Dr. Dandy with providing the inspiration he needed to develop an operative technique which he reasoned could readily have been combined with the careful neurosurgery of Drs. Cushing and Horrax, but in those days of burgeoning surgical practice, not much time could have been devoted to observation. It was largely his own ingenuity and resourcefulness which led to the development of a remarkable surgical ability.

Dr. Poppen was born in Drenthe, Michigan, on February 27, 1903. His father and mother were both of Dutch ancestry and lived on a farm which had been the family homesite. Even as a young boy he was interested in hunting and had a dog and a gun at a very early age. His mother died when he was 10 years old, but his father was a source of strength as were other members of his father's family. Several of his relatives became physicians and medical missionaries. Dr. Poppen was educated at Hope Preparatory School in Holland, Michigan, and then at Hope College, from which he later received the degree of Doctor of Science. During this time he managed to teach school for 2 years in the upper elementary grades. A hard-working student, he was also an excellent athlete, particularly in basketball and baseball. The latter sport provided a livelihood for him during summer vacations from college and early medical school, but his experiences as a professional baseball pitcher also helped in the molding of his character and thinking.

Upon graduation from Rush Medical College in 1930, he spent a year of internship at St. Luke's Hospital in Chicago before entering his residency. In April 1933 he married Nancy High, a young lady from Wyoming, whom he met in Chicago. They lived in the Boston area since July 1933 with their two children and now have two grandchildren. Through the years he continued to have an interest in baseball and became an active golfer, and hunted big game wherever it could be found.

In his 30 years of neurosurgical practice, Dr. Poppen found time to describe his enormous surgical experience in a large number of publications, culminating with his well-known *Atlas of Neurosurgical Technique*, but he was best known for his unique and exceptional operative skill. His residents and associates always marveled at his ability to accomplish what often seemed the impossible in the operating room, yet it was a mark of his character that he always treated the most minor operation or procedure with just as much care and dignity. The same challenge existed to complete a lumbar puncture accurately and painlessly as to clip an intracranial aneurysm. He demanded much of his associates and assistants and much of himself. No task was too menial; there was no patient who could not be seen, no human feeling that was not considered. His aggressiveness and capacity for work throughout his career earned him the respect, if not always the endearment, of his colleagues. His surgical approach was neither ritualistic nor fussy, but his insistence upon an orderly "chronological" sequence was the keynote of every operation. This, coupled with knowledge and judgment based upon thousands of cases, led to the development of a school of neurosurgery which was badly needed and will be long enduring.

His achievements were recognized by many awards and honors from North and South American and European institutions. He served as president of the Boston Society of Neurology and Psychiatry, the Harvey Cushing Society, and the Society of Neurological Surgeons. He was also a member of the American Neurological Association, the American Surgical Association, the Boston Surgical Society, The Massachusetts Medical Society, the American Medical Association, and was a Fellow of the American College of Surgeons. Dr. James Poppen died in 1978.

CHARLES A. FAGER, M.D.

Austin Roy Tyrer, Jr.

Dr. Austin Roy Tyrer, Jr., earned his B.S. degree at Andrews University, Berrien Springs, Michigan, in 1940, and his M.D. at Loma Linda University, Loma Linda, California, in 1944. His postgraduate training in neurosurgery (1944–50) was accomplished at Loma Linda, Lahey Clinic in Boston, and at the University of Tennessee, and included as well 2 years in the United States Army as chief of neurosurgery at Letterman General Hospital in San Francisco, California. He was certified by the American Board of Neurosurgery in 1952.

It is impossible in the space allowed to describe all the professional and civic activities to which this tireless, civic-minded professional has contributed his time, energy, and organizational talents. Likewise, it is beyond the scope of this document to list all the honors he has accumulated in his industrious lifetime. Those listed here are the ones he himself might choose as most significant.

As one of the 22 founding members of the Congress of Neurological Surgeons (CNS), Dr. Tyrer served as its 13th president. At the beginning of his presidential year, he left immediately from the Houston meeting in October 1963, on a round-the-world trip for the purpose of initiating a neurosurgical volunteer program in India. The success of this international neurosurgical exchange program in India, later Malaysia, and other developing countries, played a significant role in the establishment in 1969 of the Foundation for International Education in Neurosurgery (FIENS). A founding member, Dr. Tyrer has served on the FIENS Board since its inception, and was chairman of its Board for 16 years.

In 1964, as part of the 13th Annual CNS meeting in Denver, Colorado, Dr. Tyrer initiated the first closed-circuit color telecast of a neurosurgical operation in progress from the operating suite at Presbyterian Hospital, Denver. This was accomplished through the courtesy and cooperation of Smith, Kline & French Laboratory.

In 1990, the American Association of Neurological Surgeons honored Dr. Tyrer for his multiple international, national, state, and local services by choosing him as the fourth recipient of their Humanitarian Award. Among the contributions that this award commended were Dr. Tyrer's active membership on the American Medical Association (AMA) House of Delegates (1967–1991), his 10 years on the AMA Council on Voluntary Health Agencies (including its chairmanship), his 6 years on the AMA Council on Medical Service (an elected position), his membership on the Advisory Committee on Volunteer Physicians in Vietnam, and his 6 years on the President's Committee on Employment of the Handicapped. He has been president of the Society of Medical Consultants to the Armed Forces. He also served two tours of duty on the Good Ship Hope. The Egyptian Neurosurgical Society has accorded him honorary membership.

Dr. Tyrer has been in active private practice in Memphis, Tennessee, since 1950, having been a founding member of the partnership of Gotten, Hawkes, and Tyrer, later the Neurosurgical Group of Memphis, PA (now PC). He is clinical professor of neurosurgery at the University of Tennessee, Memphis. In Memphis, he has been president of the Medical Society, the Board of Health, the Rotary Club, the Executives' Club, and Junior Achievement. He was instrumental in having a state institution for the mentally impaired built in West Tennessee, and is a life trustee of the United Way. During his more than 40 years of neurosurgical practice, he has served as chief of neurosurgery for the Methodist Hospitals of Memphis, and in 1989 was given their Living Award. Dr. Tyrer continues to see neurosurgical patients 5 days weekly.

FLORENCE BRUCE

1964

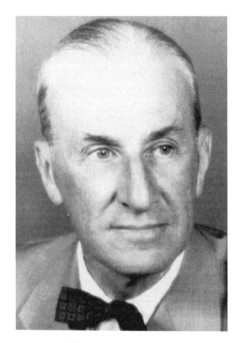

EDGAR A. KAHN

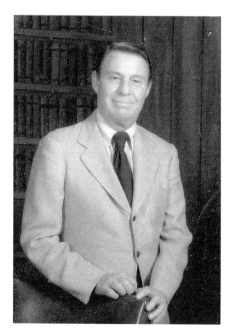

EDWARD CLINTON WEIFORD

Edgar A. Kahn

Our distinguished guest, Dr. Edgar A. Kahn, whom we honored in 1964, was held in high esteem and affection by his colleagues and by the many neurosurgeons he trained over the years at the University of Michigan. He was born in Detroit in 1900, the only son among the four children of Mr. and Mrs. Albert Kahn. As a youth he attended Andover Academy in Massachusetts, but after graduation returned to his native Midwest to enter his mother's alma mater, the University of Michigan, with which he has been associated ever since. He was elected captain of the first University of Michigan hockey team in 1923, a position which called for the physical agility, coordination, mental alertness, and endurance which are so characteristic of him. Even in 1964 one may have often found him skating on an Ann Arbor park rink with his attractive young daughters.

It is infrequent that a man internationally known in one field has a son who achieves acclaim in an entirely different field. Albert Kahn was an architect, world famous for the design of the modern assembly line factory he developed for the automobile industry. He also designed office buildings for Detroit and other cities, and many of the finest buildings on the University of Michigan campus. Although Edgar accompanied his father on business trips to Europe and Russia and spent a summer working in the firm's office, he soon realized that this was not the work in which he wished to spend the remainder of his life. He entered the Medical School at the University of Michigan and received his M.D. degree in 1924. A rotating internship and an assistant residency in general surgery under Dr. Hugh Cabot followed. In 1926 Dr. Max Minor Peet of the surgical staff decided to limit himself to the practice of neurosurgery and took on Dr. Kahn as his first resident. Thus began a close association that was to continue, with the exception of the war years, for the remainder of Dr. Peet's life. Dr. Kahn became an assistant professor in 1929, associate professor in 1934, and after Dr. Peet's death was appointed, in 1950, professor and chairman of the Section of Neurosurgery at Michigan.

Early in 1940, Dr. Kahn volunteered his services to a Red Cross Unit that was destined for France. Unfortunately, France fell before the unit could see service and its members barely escaped from Paris before the onrushing German forces. He later joined the United States Army as chief of neurosurgery of the 298th General Hospital (University of Michigan). In England he became a lieutenant colonel and chief of surgery of this unit, and later in France was the chief of a neurosurgical center at the 48th General Hospital in Paris. At the end of the war he was discharged as a colonel. Following the war he was consulting neurosurgeon at Percy Jones Veterans' Hospital in Battle Creek, Michigan and has been chief of neurosurgery at the United States Veterans' Hospital in Ann Arbor. During recent years he has been a civilian consultant in neurosurgery to the Air Force.

Early in Dr. Kahn's career he pioneered in the use of craniotomy for the removal of subdural hemotomas in infancy. He was the first surgeon to inject Thorotrast into brain abscesses, using serial x-rays to check on the localization, size, and course of the lesion. With Dr. Max Peet he was responsible for the development of bilateral supradiaphragmatic splanchnicectomy in the treatment of hypertension. Dr. Kahn did much to aid in the standardization of the technique of thoracic anterolateral cordotomy in the treatment of intractable pain. He described the dentate ligament syndrome in one of the first papers to emphasize the importance of neuroanatomical pathways within the spinal cord. The surgery of all brain tumors has always been of special interest to him, but in recent years he has been particularly interested in the challenge of the surgery of craniopharyngiomas and their preoperative and postoperative problems.

Our guest was first and foremost a clinical neurosurgeon of distinction, and although not usually an active participant in experimental research, he was always interested in its practical applications. He was instrumental in securing the internationally famous neuroanatomist, Dr. Elizabeth C. Crosby, as director of the Kresge Neurosurgical Research Laboratory at Michigan upon her retirement from active teaching in the Anatomy Department. This fostered a closer and very productive relationship between the basic science of neuroanatomy and clinical work. As senior coauthors of the book *Correlative Neurosurgery* Dr. Kahn and Dr. Crosby emphasized this cooperation through three editions.

Dr. Kahn was one of the original Diplomates of the American Board of Surgery (1937) and of the American Board of Neurological Surgery (1940) and served as a member of the latter board from 1954 through 1960. Among the societies of which he was a member are the American College of Surgeons, the Central Surgical Association, the American Neurological Association, and the French Neurosurgical Society. He was a founding member of The Harvey Cushing Society and its president in 1954. He was also a member of the Society of Neurological Surgeons and served as its president in 1957.

Anyone who knew our honored guest cannot help but be impressed with the wide variety of interests which were so much a part of his life. From his family he acquired an early appreciation of art and of French culture. For many years he was an enthusiastic pilot of his own planes. He enjoyed boating on the Great Lakes in the summer and skiing with his family in the winter.

In 1949 Dr. Kahn married the charming Rose Hermann Parker, a capable internist in her own right, and they had three attractive young daughters. The family was on a winter sabbatical in Europe in 1964. The girls were already in school in Switzerland and Dr. Kahn delayed his departure in order to be the honored guest of the Congress.

Dr. Kahn's qualities of intellectual curiosity, continuing self-criticism, and enthusiasm made him a leader in his field. His flair for the occasional unexpected and original delighted his friends. His genuine warmth and desire to aid a patient in distress, or a resident or medical student in difficulty, engendered a deep loyalty and respect in all who knew him. Dr. Edgar Kahn died August 29, 1985.

RICHARD C. SCHNEIDER, M.D.

Edward Clinton Weiford

Dr. Edward Clinton Weiford was born on July 4, 1918 in Kansas City, Missouri. He graduated from Westport High School in 1935 with varsity letters as quarterback in football, forward in basketball, and state medalist in the half-mile. He was elected to the Honor Society.

He received his A.B. degree from the University of Kansas in 1939, and graduated from the Medical School in 1942, having been elected to Alpha Omega Alpha scholastic medical fraternity in his junior year. After his internship at the University of Kansas Hospitals, he served in the Navy Medical Corps from 1943 until 1946, being awarded the Bronze Star with "V" for combat in 1944 at Okinawa. He started a fellowship in Neurological Surgery in July 1946 at the Cleveland Clinic under Dr. W. James Gardner and upon completion was appointed to the staff of the clinic until he resigned to return to Kansas City in private practice in 1951 until he retired in 1981.

Dr. Weiford married Mary Claire Gillick of Shawnee, Oklahoma in 1942. They met when he, as a medical student, and she, as a nursing student, attended an obligatory autopsy. Their only son, Thomas, was born in 1946. They have three grandchildren, Jeff, age 21; Brian, age 19; and Katie, age 14.

Dr. Weiford has been quite active in the Naval Reserve finally serving as a commanding officer of the number one-rated Volunteer Medical Reserve Company preceding his retirement as a captain in 1973. His memberships include the American Association of Neurological Surgeons, the Congress of Neurological Surgeons, the Rocky Mountain Neurosurgical Society, the Central Neuropsychiatric Association, American and Missouri Medical Associations, the Missouri and Kansas City Neurosurgical Societies, and various hospital staffs. He has served as secretary and president of the Congress of Neurological Surgeons, president of the Missouri and Kansas City Neurosurgical Societies, chief of staff of St. Margaret's Hospital, honorary director of Rockhurst College, Outman Scholarship Foundation member of the University of Kansas, director of Mercantile Regional Bank, and district chairman of Funding for St. Ann's Catholic Church.

His life-long and all-consuming passion has been golf in which at age 72, he maintains a 10 handicap at Indian Hills Country Club in Kansas City and at El Camino Country Club in Oceanside, California. If you need to find him and can't, look on the golf course.

1965

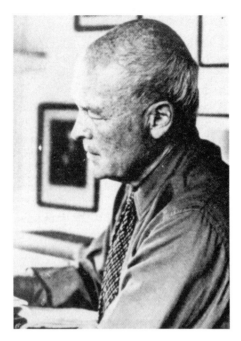

JAMES CLARKE WHITE

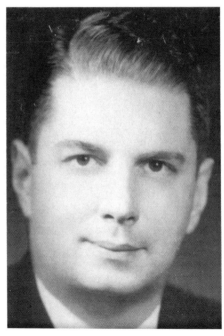

GORDON VAN DEN NOORT

James Clarke White

The career of Dr. James Clarke White was marked by a long productive period during which he devoted himself to the development of surgery of the nervous system. An early concern with the specific problems associated with intractable pain led to extensive careful exploration of measures for its relief. His continuing contributions in this field, amply emphasized by his presentations in this volume, are widely known and adopted.

Born in Austria on February 6, 1895, while his father was studying medicine in Vienna, Dr. White became a member of a family with a tradition of medicine as a career. Both his grandfather and father were professors at Harvard Medical School and chiefs of the Dermatology Department at the Massachusetts General Hospital. After graduation from Groton, Dr. White entered Harvard College and received his A.B. degree in chemistry *cum laude* in 1917. Following 2 years of Navy service as a watch and division officer on a light cruiser, he returned to Harvard and in 1923 was awarded his M.D. degree *magna cum laude*. The year 1923–1924 was spent as an intern in pathology at The Johns Hopkins Hospital. While maintaining a great interest in Dr. Harvey Cushing's work in neurosurgery, Dr. White went into general surgery and spent the years 1924–1927 at the Massachusetts General Hospital as intern and resident in general surgery. In 1927, he received a Moseley Travelling Fellowship from Harvard Medical School which enabled him to spend 6 months working on problems of the sympathetic nervous system and pain surgery with Professor A. Hovelacque in Paris and Professor René Leriche in Strasbourg.

On returning to Boston in 1928, Dr. White joined the Massachusetts General Hospital staff in general surgery, working particularly in the surgery of vascular disease and pain in cardiovascular disease. In 1935, he became a member of the neurosurgical staff and in 1941 was appointed its chief. At this time, however, he again entered the Navy, serving for 5 years in the Medical Corps as chief of neurosurgery at the United States Naval Hospitals in Chelsea, Massachusetts, and St. Albans, New York. His work at these hospitals was especially concerned with injury to the spinal cord and peripheral nerves. After discharge from active duty with the rank of captain, Dr. White returned to full-time duty at the Massachusetts General Hospital. In addition, he served the Veterans Administration for 10 years as branch section chief of neurosurgery for the New England area. During this time, he helped to supervise the organization of Veterans Administration neurosurgical facilities. Dr. White remained in the Naval Reserve until 1953 when he retired. He maintained continuing interests in riding and shooting, as well as a lifelong love for the sea.

In addition to his work as chief of neurosurgery at the Massachusetts General Hospital, Dr. White had a long teaching and research career. Beginning as alumni assistant in surgery at Harvard in 1926, he taught for an uninterrupted period of 35 years. In 1955, he was named professor of surgery of the Harvard Medical School at the Massachusetts General Hospital. As one of the outstanding teachers on the Harvard faculty, Dr. White's early and long interest in the tutorial program has been an effective stimulus in the physiological approach to surgery for many of the Medical School's students. In the training of pre- and postdoctoral fellows, he established and maintained a high standard of academic surgery.

Dr. White's investigative interests in neurosurgery were connected primarily with neurovisceral physiology and the mechanisms and relief of chronic painful conditions. These resulted in over 160 publications, including two textbooks: *The Autonomic Nervous System*, three editions, the third with Dr. R. H. Smithwick and Dr. F. A. Simeone; and *Pain: Its Mechanisms and Neurosurgical Control*, with Dr. W. H. Sweet. At the Massachusetts General Hospital, he helped to develop laboratories and fostered investigation in many diverse areas of neurosurgical research.

In 1961, Dr. White retired as chief of neurosurgery at the Massachusetts General Hospital and professor of surgery at Harvard Medical School, but he continued medical writing and maintained a private practice. His own meticulous patient records were illustrated by detailed drawings of each operative procedure. In October 1962, he gave a series of lectures at a number of Japanese universities, and in the spring of 1963 participated in the Middle East Medical Assembly, presenting the Wilder Penfield Lecture at the American University of Beirut.

Throughout his long career, Dr. White actively participated in professional societies and organizations. He was vice chairman of the American Board of Neurological Surgery, president of the Boston Society of Psychiatry and Neurology, vice president of the American Neurological Association, and a member of the National Institutes of Health Study Section on Neurology. He was also a member of the American Surgical Association, the American Medical Association, the Harvey Cushing Society, the Association for Research in Nervous and Mental Disease, the American College of Surgeons, the Society of Neurological Surgeons, the Boston Surgical Society, and the American Academy of Arts and Sciences. Internationally, Dr. White was a member of the Académie de Chirurgie (Paris), the Société de Chirurgie de Lyon, the International Society of Surgery, and an honorary member of the Société de Neurochirurgie de Langue Français. Dr. James White died in January 1981.

ROBERT G. OJEMANN, M.D.

Gordon van den Noort

Gordon van den Noort was born May 8, 1922 in Buitenzorg, Java, Netherlands East Indies, of American parents. He attended Dartmouth College and graduated in November, 1943 with a B.A. degree. He then attended the Temple University School of Medicine and received his M.D. Degree in 1947. He interned at the Philadelphia General Hospital in 1947 to 1948 and was a resident in neurology at Philadelphia General Hospital in 1948 to 1949. He then was a resident in neurological surgery at the Graduate Hospital of the University of Pennsylvania under the direction of Dr. Robert Groff in 1949 to 1953. This residency was interrupted by a 21-month term as captain in the Army Medical Corps. During that time he served as assistant chief of the neurosurgical section at the Valley Forge Army Hospital. After Dr. van den Noort completed his

residency in neurological surgery he became Dr. Groff's assistant and associated with Dr. Groff from July 1953 to November 1956. He then entered
private practice in Bryn Mawr, Pennsylvania.

Dr. van den Noort served as treasurer of the Congress of Neurological Surgeons (CNS) between 1960 and 1963 and became president of the CNS in 1965.
He was appalled to discover that the day after he was inducted into office that
he was expected to give a presidential address the following day. The result
was an address that was notable for its brevity. He felt strongly that the
presidential address should be delivered at the end of the term and he was
successful in implementing this reform the following year when Dr. Mosberg,
Dr. van den Noort's successor, was stuck with two presidential addresses, one
on each end of his term.

Dr. van den Noort in his brief presidential address made the first appeal for
cooperation between the Congress of Neurological Surgeons and the American
Association of Neurological Surgeons. Dr. van den Noort was very pleased to
see the mutual effort that evolved between these two fine organizations. Dr.
van den Noort was appointed to the Board of Directors of the American Association of Neurological Surgeons (AANS) as Representative of the Congress.
At that time the AANS had a representative from the major neurosurgical
societies. Dr. van den Noort became treasurer of the AANS in 1968 and served
in that capacity until 1970. He then was secretary from 1971 to 1974.

Dr. van den Noort was a member of the Council of the Pennsylvania Neurosurgical Society from 1980 to 1985 and president of the Mid-Atlantic Neurosurgical Society in 1982. Dr. van den Noort continued in the private practice
of neurological surgery in Bryn Mawr and Abington, Pennsylvania until his
retirement in 1983.

1966

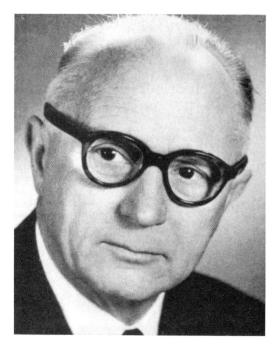

Hugo A. Krayenbühl

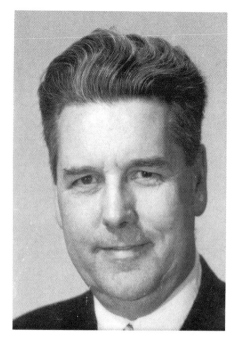

William H. Mosberg, Jr.

Hugo A. Krayenbühl

Neurological surgery as it exists in Switzerland today owes its high level of competence to its founder, Professor Hugo A. Krayenbühl. Coming to neurosurgery from a background of neurology, surgery, and psychiatry, he was the only holder of the professorship in neurosurgery at the University of Zürich and was the head of the neurosurgical service at the University Hospital in Zürich.

The son of a physician, Dr. Krayenbühl was born in Zihlschlacht, Switzerland, on December 3, 1902. After attending the university at St. Gallen, he studied medicine in Geneva, Kiel, Paris, and Zürich. Upon the acceptance of his dissertation, "Beitrag zur Kenntnis der Ewing'schen Knochensarkome," by the University of Zürich in 1928, he became a Doctor of Medicine.

His postgraduate studies led him to pathology, internal medicine, and then to neurology and psychiatry. After receiving his neurological training at the Charité, Berlin, under the outstanding German neurologist, Geheimrat Professor Karl Bonhoeffer, he studied psychiatry under Professor C. Maier at the world-famous Psychiatric University Clinic Burghölzli in Zürich. Observing the poor results obtained by European surgeons in treating tumors of the brain, Dr. Krayenbühl became interested in neurosurgery and, in preparation for his entrance into this new field, he took several months of training in general surgery in Zürich.

From 1934 to 1936, Dr. Krayenbühl worked in London under Sir Hugh Cairns, the eminent pupil of Harvey Cushing. Through Dr. Cairns he became familiar with the techniques of Dr. Cushing and the traditions of the Cushing school. Because of the influence of Dr. Cairns, Professor Krayenbühl remained deeply attached to British neurology and neurosurgery.

Upon his return to Zürich in 1936, Dr. Krayenbühl was given the opportunity to work at the University Clinic and to build his own department of neurosurgery. The Kanton Zürich offered the necessary accommodations, but only on the condition that Dr. Krayenbühl himself provide table, lighting, instruments, and an x-ray unit for the operating theater. The first operation took place on July 13, 1936. From these small beginnings, the Clinic grew, and, through his devotion, efficiency, and high standards, Dr. Krayenbühl became known as the leading neurosurgeon in Switzerland. In 1939 the Clinic was officially recognized as an independent unit, and in 1948 Professor Krayenbühl was given the first chair of neurosurgery in Switzerland by the University of Zürich. In 1966, his neurosurgical Clinic had 76 beds, between 1,800 and 1,900 admissions each year, and 16 clinical assistants. On May 23, 1966, the 20,000th operation took place.

In addition to his devotion to his patients and to the Clinic, Professor Krayenbühl was deeply concerned with the teaching of students and the training of neurosurgeons working at his Clinic. In Switzerland, the directors of the neurosurgical university clinics of Basel, Geneva, and Lausanne, of the neurological university clinics of Basel and Berne, and of the encephalographic department at Lausanne are his former pupils. Many distinguished neurosurgeons from other countries also took their specialized training under him.

Through his research and publications, Dr. Krayenbühl made valuable contributions to the field of neurosurgery. Since 1941, when his "Habilitations-schrift" on the aneurysm of the brain was published, he was concerned with disturbances of cerebral circulation. He published important papers on cerebral venous, carotid, and vertebral thrombosis and on spasms of the cerebral arteries. His endeavors in the field of diagnostic and therapeutic problems of aneurysms of the brain culminated in the publication of *The Cerebral Angiography* in 1965 with M. G. Yasargil. The total number of his published books and papers exceeded 150 in 1966.

Professor Krayenbühl drew strength and support for his manifold activities from the lively circle of his family. Since 1933 he was married to Elsa Gross, L.D. They had one daughter and three sons. His understanding, amiable, and wise wife shared with him a love for music, modern painting, and sculpture which counterbalanced the strain of his professional duties. Intuitive, far seeing, decisive, and with a joy in the precision of his skill, Dr. Krayenbühl himself was, indeed, a rare combination of the artist and craftsman.

The power of his single-minded concentration on so many activities brought Dr. Krayenbühl well deserved recognition and honor. He was an honorary member or fellow of many European and American neurological and neurosurgical societies. He was the president of the First European Congress for Neurosurgery, which was held in Zürich in 1959. In 1966, Professor Krayenbühl was 64 years old and was full of youthful energy, vividly responding to new ideas, planning ahead for the future of his clinic and of the University. Dr. Hugo Krayenbühl died in 1985.

GERHARD WEBER, M.D.

William H. Mosberg, Jr.

William H. Mosberg, Jr. was born on August 22, 1920 in Baltimore, Maryland. His early education was in Baltimore public schools. He graduated from high school in 1936 at the age of 15, in the midst of the Depression and there was no money for college. He enrolled in business college from which he graduated within 1 year with a proficiency in shorthand and typing both of which he continues to use regularly. After working in an iron foundry for 1 year, he began his premedical studies at the University of Maryland. After graduating from the University of Maryland School of Medicine, internship and residency training were completed at the University of Maryland Hospital. He completed the neurosurgical residency program at that institution in 1949 including 2 years as a captain in the Army of the United States in the European Theater of Operations. There followed 1 year in neurology at the National Hospital, Queen's Square; brief periods at the Radcliffe Infirmary, Oxford in neurosurgery; Hospital de la Salpetriere, Paris in neurology; and then Mercy Hospital, Loyola University Clinics, Chicago in neurosurgery. After 1 year of research in neurophysiology at the Illinois Neuropsychiatric Institute, Chicago and the Department of Electrical Engineering, Champaign-Urbana, he returned to the faculty of the University of Maryland School of Medicine and the private practice of neurosurgery in Baltimore.

Through the intervening 4 decades, Dr. Mosberg has fulfilled many committee assignments; only committee chairmanships and elected offices will be mentioned. He was chairman of the Editorial Committee of the Congress of Neurological Surgeons (CNS) and editor-in-chief of *Clinical Neurosurgery* for the 1960, 1961, and 1962 meetings. In 1963 he was the first chairman of a CNS Socio-Economics Committee. In that capacity, he initiated the *Neurosurgical Fee Survey* publication for which a CNS Distinguished Service Award was subsequently granted. He was appointed chairman of the Scientific Program Committee for the 1964 annual meeting. Therefore, the completion of the *Neurosurgical Fee Survey* was turned over to Dr. Edward Bishop, the recipient of the Distinguished Service Award.

Dr. Mosberg was elected president of the Congress of Neurological Surgeons for the 1965–1966 year. It was customary at that time for the newly elected president to give his presidential address upon assuming office. A major event in United States neurosurgery at that time was the recent proclamation by Dr. Frank Mayfield as president of the then Harvey Cushing Society that that organization should be the "spokesman for neurosurgery." Dr. Mosberg's presidential address upon assuming office had to do with the decision of the Executive Committee in this matter and was entitled "The Affirmation of a Proclamation." Subsequently, he represented the CNS on the Ad Hoc Liaison Committee to formulate the reorganization of our specialty. It was in this decade that United States neurosurgery became intensely involved in international neurosurgery. A "visiting professor" type of program involving the Christian Medical College, Vellore, South India, was funded by the Office of Vocational Rehabilitation, Department of Health, Education and Welfare. This office also funded programs in Pakistan and Egypt. Dr. Mosberg was a participant visiting India, Pakistan, and Egypt prior to and again immediately following his tenure as president of the Congress. He was appointed representative of the Congress to *CARE MEDICO* in 1962 and served in that capacity as neurosurgical advisor to *CARE-MEDICO* for the next 2 decades when such overseas activities by *CARE-MEDICO* were terminated. During those years, he visited and participated in overseas programs in South Vietnam, Malaysia, Ceylon, Indonesia, Afghanistan, Tunisia, Algeria, Jordan, Dominican Republic, and Haiti. From 1972 to 1980 he was chairman of the Professional Committee and a member of the Executive Committee and Corporate Board of *CARE-MEDICO*. He had served in 1964 on the CNS Ad Hoc Head Injury Nomenclature Committee. In 1966 as president of the CNS he appointed (and served on) the committee producing a *Glossary of Neurosurgical Operative Procedure Nomenclature*. As president of the CNS he proposed and implemented the concept of the Distinguished Service Award of the CNS, and also proposed and appointed a committee to assemble the publication *Utilization Guidelines*, for which Dr. Walter Lockhart received the Distinguished Service Award. During his year as president of the CNS he proposed and developed plans to implement the formation of the Foundation for International Education in Neurological Surgery. During the 1965 to 1966 year, the Executive Committee of the CNS decreed that the president of the CNS should give his presidential address at the end of his term in office. For his second presidential address, Dr. Mosberg discussed his proposal for an international educational foundation. There has been continuing involvement in international neuro-surgical education and in socio-economic affairs as they relate to neurosurgery. He served as secretary of the Foundation for International Education in Neu-rological Surgery from the inception of that organization in 1969 until he resigned from that office in 1991. He was appointed chairman of the Committee on Neurosurgical Education of the World Federation of Neurosurgical Societies in 1973 and editor of *Federation News* in 1982, and served in both capacities until he resigned in 1989. He has also served as chairman of a number of committees of the American Association of Neurological Surgeons (AANS) including International Affairs Committee (1976–1981), Committee on For-eign Neurosurgical Training (1976–1982), Adjunct Committee on correspond-ing Members (1975–1984), Coordinating Committee (1972–1973), and By Laws Committee (1974–1975). In the area of socio-economic affairs, he has been a member of the Joint Socio-Economic Committee (subsequently the Joint Coun-cil of State Neurosurgical Societies) since its inception in 1972 and chairman of its International Committee from 1975 until his resignation in 1990. He has been editor for Socio-economic Perspectives of *Neurosurgery* since 1978. From 1967 to 1969, he was Chairman of an ad hoc committee of the CNS to effect affiliation between the Congress of Neurological Surgeons and the In-terurban Neurosurgical Society. He has been a member of the Board of Di-rectors of the Interurban Neurosurgical Society since 1969.

Dr. Mosberg was a member of the Editorial Board of the *Bulletin of the School of Medicine, University of Maryland* from 1957 to 1970, and of *The American Surgeons* from 1963 to 1988. He was elected president of the medical staff of Maryland General Hospital from 1962 to 1964 and held the same office at the University of Maryland Hospital from 1968 to 1969 and at Saint Joseph Hospital from 1976 to 1978. He was elected secretary, Maryland Chapter, of the American College of Surgeons from 1961 to 1966. He served as president of the Medical Alumni Association, University of Maryland from 1975 to 1976. He was a delegate from the American Medical Association to the Third World Conference on Medical Education, New Delhi, India in 1966. Dr. Mosberg's initial faculty appointment at the School of Medicine, University of Maryland was that of instructor in 1952. He advanced up through the ranks until he was appointed clinical professor in 1973. He held that rank until 1990 when he was promoted to emeritus clinical professor.

Dr. Mosberg retired from the clinical practice of neurological surgery in 1987, and within a short time, took a full-time job with the Federal government as chief of the branch of the Social Security Administration having to do with surgical disability claims.

1967

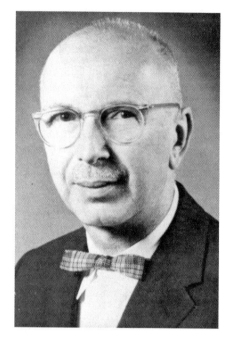

W. James Gardner

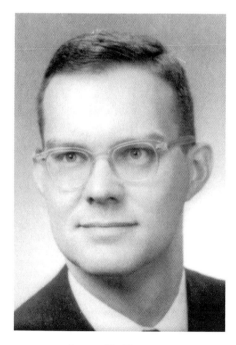

John R. Russell

W. James Gardner

Two unforeseen events helped to shape and direct the career of W. James Gardner, M.D., the honored guest of the Seventeenth Annual Meeting of the Congress of Neurological Surgeons. Suffice it to say, however, that Dr. Gardner is a man who would have had an illustrious career in any field of endeavor, regardless of circumstances.

The first and perhaps more important of these two events was the one that led to his decision to become a neurosurgeon rather than follow in the footsteps of his father who was a general surgeon in McKeesport, Pennsylvania. After receiving his M.D. degree in 1924, Dr. Gardner remained at the University of Pennsylvania School of Medicine for training which was to include 2 years of internship and 3 years of general surgery. Each intern was required to spend 3 months on the service of Charles H. Frazier, M.D., professor of surgery and head of the division of surgery. Dr. Frazier limited his surgery mainly to neurological and thyroid problems. An autocrat both in and out of the surgical amphitheatre, he was a perfectionist who operated meticulously and would not tolerate the slightest blood loss. The Frazier service was not well liked by the house staff because of the long, arduous hours and the stern demeanor of its chief. Just as Dr. Gardner began his tour of duty with Dr. Frazier, the resident resigned and full responsibility for running the service fell on Dr. Gardner, the intern. At the end of 3 months, since no resident had been found, Dr. Gardner stayed on for a second period out of sympathy for Dr. Frazier's predicament. Somewhere during this period a spark was struck that ignited his interest in neurosurgery, because plans for training in general surgery were discarded in favor of neurosurgery. Our honored guest remained with Dr. Frazier for a further 3 years, thus formalizing his training in neurosurgery, a field that he probably would not have entered if he had not been exposed to such an unexpectedly intensive beginning. One of the highlights of these formative years, according to Dr. Gardner's recollection, was the frequent consultations between Dr. Frazier and the noted Philadelphia neurologist Dr. W. G. Spiller.

The second happenstance to alter Dr. Gardner's life was the Cleveland Clinic disaster in May 1929, which took the lives of 126 persons, including that of its neurosurgeon, Charles E. Locke, M.D. Instead of returning to the Pittsburgh area as he had contemplated, Dr. Gardner, on the recommendation of Dr. Frazier, joined the staff of the Cleveland Clinic to fill the unexpected opening. Thus began a most fruitful and rewarding association which was to last for 35 years.

Dr. Gardner wrote more than 200 scientific papers. For the most part his contributions were clinically oriented, since he was not one to pursue a laboratory project for the sake of pure science. There must be some clinical application to each bit of experimental work, or he paid it scant attention. He always maintained that there was nothing more stimulating to a curious mind than the problems encountered in the care of sick patients. A constant source of amazement to his resident staff was his ability to recall and apply effectively experimental evidence in order to explain clinical phenomena and solve clinical problems.

Despite an extremely active surgical and outpatient practice, Dr. Gardner was never without some project to further occupy his time. Each problem was followed through with dogged determination even though the initial results may have been enough to discourage the most enthusiastic participant. Inventiveness and serendipity, combined with hard work and determination, were among his greatest attributes. Although the work for the resident staff seemed endless, not one on his service could say that he worked harder than "the boss."

Because his interests were so numerous and varied, it was difficult to select the outstanding contribution that Dr. Gardner made to the specialty of neurosurgery. A large surgical practice made it imperative for him to develop surgical techniques that were quick, effective, without frills, and advantageous for patient and surgeon. He was one of the early proponents of the sitting position for both cranial and spinal surgery. From this developed the use of the "G suit" to control venous pressure and prevent air embolism. In addition, he developed a surgical chair with such versatility that it could be utilized with the patient in any position and a head clamp for positive fixation of the skull during surgery. He was the first to advocate and use induced arterial hypotension for intracranial surgery.

Neurological and roentgenographic diagnosis occupied much of Dr. Gardner's attention over the years. An excellent neurologist, he always found that neurological problems present a challenge, even though not of a surgical nature. He was among the first to advocate the use of pneumoencephalography for the diagnosis of suspected intracranial surgical problems, even when these were associated with increased intracranial pressure. The procedure of lumbar discography was quickly adopted and he used it successfully for more than 15 years.

The six papers that he wrote on chronic subdural hematoma, which include the first satisfactory explanation of the so-called latent interval and an effective method of reexpanding the cerebral hemisphere after drainage of a chronic subdural hematoma, were evidence of Dr. Gardner's interest in this subject. His vast experience in the management of tic douloureux, a major interest throughout his career, was concerned not only with treatment but also with the development of a theory of the pathophysiology of this condition.

Since 1950, when our honored guest first wrote about the surgical treatment of Arnold-Chiari malformation, he devoted considerable time and effort to the study of this and related problems. Gradually there evolved a theory of the common origin of such conditions as Arnold-Chiari malformation, Dandy-Walker syndrome, syringomyelia, meningomyelocele, and certain forms of congenital hydrocephalus. While this idea was by no means universally accepted, the concept was exciting and it challenged the somewhat rigid theories of the time.

Wartime service in the Navy introduced him to the use of Tantalum for cranioplasty. He continued to use it since that time and advocated immediate repair of cranial defects with Tantalum, even in the presence of compound wounds.

Total care of the patient was always Dr. Gardner's goal and custom. He maintained that the patient suffers when the responsibility for management is divided among two services or more. This concern in his inventive mind led to the development of a number of interesting devices to ensure proper patient care. Perhaps the best known of these is the alternating pressure pad which applies a pneumatic principle in the prevention and treatment of bedsores.

His pioneering work was manifested in several other areas, namely, cerebral hemispherectomy in the treatment of glioma, the treatment of carotid cavernous fistula by muscle embolization, the application of sympathectomy in the treatment of various ailments, the surgical treatment of hemifacial spasm, and the use of intraspinal steroid injections in the treatment of sciatica.

The ability and willingness to teach were always among Dr. Gardner's greatest attributes. He liked nothing better than to show an exhibit at a medical meeting, where he could be found from opening to closing time hard at work explaining his theories and observations to an interested audience. Over the years there was a steady procession of residents passing through his service. By 1967, Dr. Gardner had given full training to 28 neurosurgeons and partial training to 14 others, not to mention the innumerable general surgical residents who spent a few months in neurosurgery. Each man was always given the opportunity to work, study, and participate to the best of his ability. He could feel secure in the knowledge that the Chief would give him full backing and support both during his training and thereafter.

Dr. Gardner was born in McKeesport, Pennsylvania, on June 12, 1898. He attended Washington and Jefferson College (A.B. 1920). He received his M.D. from the University of Pennsylvania Medical School in 1924, as did his father, William James, 30 years before, and his son, William James III, 30 years later. He had a fond attachment to western Pennsylvania where he spent many of his boyhood summers hunting and fishing in the Allegheny forests and streams.

Dr. Gardner maintained his interest in outdoor activities throughout his life. He had a particular fondness for hunting, and managed to indulge in this hobby despite his active schedule. He participated in sports with the same zeal and energy that was given to scientific pursuits, and remained a prime protagonist of all physical culture. He took up ice skating and tennis at the age of 50 and did well with both sports. His skiing career, however, ended with a broken tibia. An excellent dancer, he thoroughly enjoyed a party, where he probably was found sometime during the occasion busily organizing and participating in a bit of "close barbershop harmony."

Dr. Gardner was married to Ann Ray Kieffer of San Angelo, Texas, and had three children, including W. James III, a general surgeon in Utah. During World War I, he served in the United States Army Infantry as a private, and was a lieutenant commander in the Navy during World War II.

Dr. Gardner was active in many of the national and sectional organizations. He was president of the Society of Neurological Surgeons, vice president of the Cushing Society, and on the Board of Governors of the American College of Surgeons. He was on the Board of Neurological Surgery for 6 years. During his 35 years at the Cleveland Clinic, he served actively in many important capacities. He thoroughly believed in and enjoyed this type of group practice. Upon reaching the compulsory retirement age of 65, he entered private practice. Dr. W. James Gardner died in January 1986.

DONALD F. DOHN, M.D.

John R. Russell

John R. Russell was born March 17, 1922 in Bloomington, Indiana. The delivery of five babies that day swamped the medical staff of the town's tiny hospital, so John's father was pressed into service to administer chloroform to his parturient wife. John attended the laboratory high school of the University of Chicago, and there met his fellow editor of the school newspaper, Jane Bureau. Continuing his education at the University of Chicago, John received the degrees of B.S. in 1941, M.S. (in physiology) in 1942, and M.D. in 1945. Dr. Russell and Jane were married in 1943. Their first son was born in 1945. A son was born in 1947 and daughters born in 1953 and 1966 completed the family.

Internship, at Chicago Memorial Hospital, brought John under the spell of a great teacher and neurosurgeon, Dr. Paul C. Bucy. Neurosurgery then became Dr. Russell's quest. He next spent 2 years in military service, assigned to the Dayton, Ohio Veterans Administration Hospital. He first did general and orthopedic surgery. He then spent 1 year on the neurosurgical service organized by Dr. William E. Hunt, under the supervision of Dr. Nathaniel Hollister and Dr. Thomas Weaver. There followed 2 years of neurosurgical residency under Dr. Paul Bucy at Chicago Memorial Hospital with neuropathology tutelage by Dr. Percival Bailey. A final year of residency under Drs. Semmes and Murphey in Memphis was completed in 1951. Dr. Russell then joined Dr. Robert Heimburger on the full-time faculty of Indiana University School of Medicine in Indianapolis. They trained the school's present neurosurgical head, Dr. Robert Campbell.

Dr. Russell joined the Congress of Neurological Surgeons shortly after its founding in 1951. Early on he chaired the Survey and Placement committees. Later he served as chairman of the Scientific Program Committee. He was secretary of the Congress from 1962 to 1965, and president from 1966 to 1967. He also served on the Board of Directors of the American Association of Neurological Surgeons from 1967 to 1970.

In 1959, Dr. Russell switched to part-time teaching at Indiana University's Medical School. He went into neurosurgical practice with Dr. Charles Cure. In 1971 he became associated with Dr. Julius Goodman. The practice grew to include eight neurosurgeons by the time Dr. Russell retired in 1984. Dr. Russell and Jane retired to the shores of a beautiful lake in northern Wisconsin, the site of summer vacations since 1949. A minimum of consulting work does not interfere with a physically active life which includes swimming, cross-country skiing, and woodworking.

1968

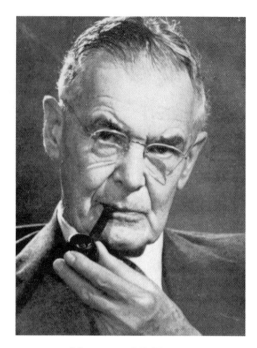

Norman M. Dott

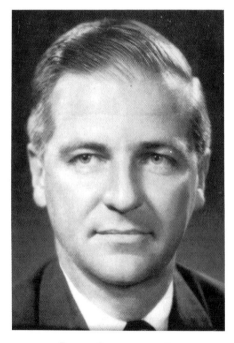

John Shillito, Jr.

Norman M. Dott

Of Scottish-Huguenot descent, Norman McOmish Dott, our distinguished guest of honor in 1968, was born in Edinburgh in 1897. His story is a romantic one; grandson and son of famous art dealers, he intended to become an engineer, but, while he was still an apprentice, a motorcycle accident caused a serious hip injury necessitating a prolonged period in the hospital. Our guest was a fascinated patient and was so intrigued by hospital activities that he decided, upon recovery, to become a medical student, and, in 1919, he graduated M.B, Ch.B. from the University of Edinburgh. He had volunteered for military service but was turned down on medical grounds. This was an added challenge and an incentive to overcome his own disability and to help the afflicted, and, indeed, in World War II he was to establish the famous Brain Injury Unit in Bangour Hospital near Edinburgh and to be appointed consultant neurosurgeon to the Army in Scotland.

After qualifying, he underwent a period of training in general surgery and gained the fellowship of the Royal College of Surgeons of Edinburgh in 1923. During this period he was also actively engaged in original experimental physiological work on gastric secretion and on the thyroid and pituitary glands, and for his notable work on the pituitary gland he was awarded a Rockefeller Travelling Fellowship which enabled him to study in Boston under Harvey Cushing during 1923 and 1924. He was greatly impressed by the developing specialty of neurological surgery and returned to Edinburgh very enthusiastic and determined to introduce and develop this specialty. There were, however, many hurdles to be overcome and many challenges to be met, and indeed one may quote R. L. Stevenson's words, "Am I no a bonny fighter?"

He made important contributions to general and pediatric surgery, and he began to practice neurosurgery privately, because this specialty was not yet accepted in the Edinburgh hospitals. He was an indefatigable campaigner with a remarkable independence of thought and of action, and he was always very ably supported and encouraged by his charming wife, Peggy. Meticulous in all that he did, he showed, without affectation, great originality and expertise in diagnosis and in the operating room and had great sympathy for the sick and a real regard for their anxious families. Loyal service from his juniors and associates was expected and received, and, although always courteous, helpful, and a good listener, he was a strict disciplinarian who never spared himself and expected the same very high standards from his assistants. With tremendous drive, enterprise, and perspicacity, he developed the most comprehensive department of surgical neurology in the United Kingdom and, by his clinical teaching and precept, attracted doctors, nurses, and others from every part of the world to come to study and train in Edinburgh. Many of these are now very distinguished specialists in the United Kingdom and in all parts of the world.

Norman Dott had a remarkable breadth of interest in the entire field of medicine and made a great number of outstanding original contributions, in particular to surgical neurology, but also to many allied specialties and to medicine as a whole, from the clinical, administrative, teaching, and research points of view. He helped to develop anesthesia in Edinburgh from 1918 to

1920, and introduced intratracheal techniques. He made original important contributions concerning the embryology of the bowel. In 1929, using sodium iodide, he was the first person in the United Kingdom to demonstrate an arteriovenous malformation of the brain by angiography. In March 1932, using Thorotrast,* he performed the first angiogram in the United Kingdom to show a saccular intracranial aneurysm. His first vertebral angiogram was done in 1946 to demonstrate an arteriovenous malformation on a posterior cerebral artery. Another very important achievement was the 1931 operation in which he treated an aneurysm on the proximal part of a middle cerebral artery in a patient by wrapping the lesion with crushed muscle. Amongst other original clinical research activities were studies on congenital dislocation of the hip, cleft palate, cerebrospinal fluid circulation and its pathology, brain displacements and related cerebral ischemia, spinal cord compression, facial pain, the treatment of facial paralysis by extrapetrous nerve graft, and the use of hypothermia in cerebral surgery. He invented many instruments and pieces of surgical apparatus, from bowel clamps to operating tables, and designed operating theatres.

In 1947, he was appointed to the first chair of neurological surgery in the University of Edinburgh, and, on reaching the age of 65 years, when regulation required him to retire from the National Health Service and the University, he was appointed emeritus professor. He became a member of the Society of British Neurological Surgeons in 1926 and was president from 1938 to 1945. From 1955 to 1967 he was vice president of the Royal College of Surgeons of Edinburgh, and from 1966 he was the representative of that College on the General Medical Council in the United Kingdom. He rapidly gained an international reputation and has been honored by medical societies and many other scientific and learned bodies throughout the world, including the Society of Neurological Surgeons, the American Association of Neurological Surgeons (the former Harvey Cushing Society), and he was appointed a member of the Editorial Advisory Board of the *Journal of Neurosurgery* in 1968. In 1936, he was elected to Fellowship of the Royal Society of Edinburgh and in 1968 was made an honorary fellow of that Society. For his important work in surgical neurology for H. M. Forces in the 1939 to 1944 War, he was awarded the high honor of Commander of the Most Noble Order of the British Empire (C. B. E.). In 1960, he was elected president of the Scottish Association of Occupational Therapists and, in 1966, president of the Scottish Society of the History of Medicine. He was made an honorary member of the American Neurological Association in 1965, and in 1966 was elected honorary president of the World Federation of Neurosurgical Societies. Other distinctions included the Syme Surgical Fellowship, the Liston Memorial Jubilee Prize for advances in neurological surgery, and the Sir Victor Horsley Memorial Award and Lectureship.

His was indeed a great success story, and he served his specialty, his medical school, and his country with notable distinction. A particular feature was his great humanity, which was shown in many ways, for example, by helping

---

*Thorotrast, thorium dioxide, Fellows—Testagar Division, Fellows Medical Mfg. Co., Inc., Detroit, Mich.

several European medical refugees who were involved in the holocaust of the 1930s, and by his intense interest in the rehabilitation and resettlement of his patients, and by most assiduous follow-up studies. One of the honors that he must have particularly cherished was that given in 1962 when he was made a Freeman of his native city of Edinburgh. Characteristically, in his address on that occasion, he referred to the great cooperation that he had always received from his patients and to their unfaltering courage and their implicit faith in him. It is interesting that the photo-portrait included in this book was taken by one of his old patients, a lady on whom he operated in 1929 for a pituitary adenoma.

In his retirement, Norman Dott was very active in many fields, among them medical administration, medical education, and medical charitable activities, particularly in the spheres of epilepsy, paraplegia, spina bifida, and cancer. He served on several important scientific and government bodies and was always in demand as a lecturer.

Even so, he still made time for other interests which he retained all his life, in particular, fishing, especially in fast-flowing Scottish streams, and in world travel, music, and photography. He spent time with his wife, daughter and son-in-law, and his three granddaughters.

Thus we had a remarkable man, the doyen of British neurosurgeons, a man who became a legend in his own lifetime.

> "May health and peace, in mutual rays,
> shine on the evening o' his days."
> *Robert Burns*

Norman Dott died in April 1974.

PHILLIP HARRIS, F.R.C.S.E., F.R.C.P.E., F.R.S.ED.

John Shillito, Jr.

John Shillito was born in Cincinnati, Ohio in 1922. He moved to Boston in 1929 and his schooling from there on was in that area. He was a freshman at Harvard College when the Japanese attacked Pearl Harbor. Already in the Naval R.O.T.C., he continued college with that unit which was technically declared on active duty to keep its members from being drafted. During college, he did part-time work at the nearby Polaroid Corporation, which was involved in several defense contracts, and volunteered as a night orderly at the Massachusetts General Hospital.

Before college was finished, the R.O.T.C. unit was called up and Dr. Shillito was assigned to the new 2200-ton destroyer U.S.S. Brush DD 745, in early 1944. The next 2 years were spent with the carrier task forces in the Pacific where he served as a line officer in various divisions, finishing as communication officer. On return after the war, it was necessary to finish a few courses at Harvard during which time he worked with a classmate in a photography business and became interested in medicine. After adding a few premedical courses, he was able to enter Harvard Medical School in 1948 and graduated with the class of 1952. Internship was in surgery at the Peter Bent Brigham Hospital. During almost 3 years of general surgery, there were two rotations through neurosurgery not only the Brigham but also at the Children's Hospital. Experiences on that service, then under the direction of Drs. Franc Ingraham and Donald Matson, led to the change to neurosurgery in 1955.

Dr. Shillito met Bunny Hubbard who was then a secretary for cardiac surgeon Dwight Harken at the Brigham Hospital, and they were married in February 1957, during the chief residency year. That July, Dr. Shillito began 1 year in Memphis, Tennessee where he gained a wealth of adult patient experience, particularly in trauma and carotid endarterectomies under Francis Murphey at the John Gaston Hospital. In July 1958, John returned to Boston to join Drs. Ingraham and Matson on the neurosurgical attending staff at the Children's and Brigham Hospitals, where he has remained to this time.

After a stint on the Executive Committee of the Congress, and as editor of *Clinical Neurosurgery*, he became president in 1968. Norman Dott was the delightful guest of honor that year and the meeting was held in Toronto. During that year, the Congress sought and was granted representation on the Board of Governors of the American College of Surgeons. Dr. Shillito was elected to serve as that first representative and served for 3 years. He has also served on the American Board of Neurological Surgery from 1972 to 1977, was vice president of the Neurosurgical Society of America from 1971 to 1972, and later was president of the Society of Neurological Surgeons from 1982 to 1983. He served on the Board of Directors of the American Association of Neurological Surgeons from 1970 to 1973.

In 1981 Dr. Shillito published, with the help of Harvey Cushing's former artist, Mildred Codding, the *Atlas of Pediatric Neurosurgical Operations* which had been conceived of and begun by Dr. Donald Matson prior to his untimely death in 1969.

Dr. Shillito's practice has always been both pediatric and adult neurosurgery. At this writing, he is still working at least 80 hours per week!

1969

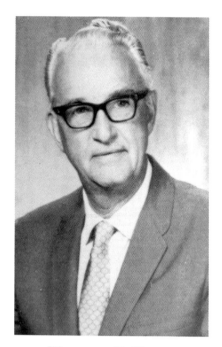

WALLACE B. HAMBY

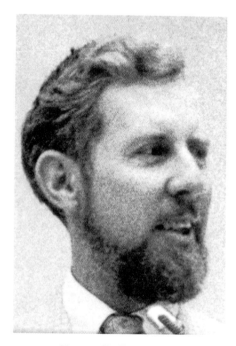

PAUL C. SHARKEY

Wallace B. Hamby

An early interest in vascular problems related to the central nervous system was evidenced by our honored guest's first medical paper, written in 1933 while he was still a resident at the Cleveland Clinic. He and his chief, Dr. W. James Gardner, published an account of their efforts to control pulsating exophthalmos due to carotid-cavernous fistulas. In this paper they reported the first successful intracranial ligation of the carotid artery.

Dr. Hamby had been attracted to the Cleveland Clinic because of its surgical renown. Although initially on the general surgical service, he soon felt an interest in the developing field of neurosurgery, and he became the Clinic's first neurosurgical resident. His training period (1929–1934) included time spent at the University of Chicago studying neuropathology.

Upon completion of his preparation, Dr. Hamby returned to Buffalo, where he had served his internship at the City Hospital, and established the Department of Neurosurgery at the University of Buffalo. After consulting at a number of hospitals, he confined most of his efforts to the Buffalo General and the Buffalo Children's Hospitals. He was professor of neurosurgery at the University of Buffalo for almost 20 years and, for a time, professor of neurology as well. He developed the department and training program into a center with an international reputation.

In 1960, our honored guest answered a call from the Cleveland Clinic to return as head of the Department of Neurological Surgery. Here he continued his interest in the teaching of neurosurgery, and, all told, more than 25 men have had part or all of their training under his tutelage.

The interest which led to his pioneering efforts in the surgical treatment of intracranial vascular lesions has continued to occupy his attention throughout his career. By 1969, he had authored 21 papers on various aspects of intracranial vascular problems. He also wrote two books on the subject, one of which, *Intracranial Aneurysms*, became a standard reference text for neurosurgeons and related specialists throughout the world.

Dr. Hamby is a master surgical technician who makes the difficult seem routine. The ease and skill with which he accomplishes surgery are perhaps a reflection in part of an artistic talent which is also manifest in his hobbies of painting, drawing, and carving. The development of new operative techniques and instruments has always been an important phase of his surgical achievement; in fact, 13 of his papers have been concerned with this area of endeavor.

Our honored guest has also made important contributions to the treatment of tic douloureux, intervertebral disc protrusions, spinal cord tumors, intractable pain, and involuntary movement disorders. He elucidated the clinical features of surgical air embolism and described a successful method of treatment.

Medical history, particularly the development of surgery, has been an avocation for him. He has followed the trail of Ambroise Paré, even to the extent of taking motor trips throughout France in pursuit of knowledge of the man and his times. Dr. Hamby is an authority on Paré, having written three books about him: *The Case Reports and Autopsy Records of Ambroise Paré, Surgery and Ambroise Paré*, and *Ambroise Paré: Surgeon of the Renaissance*.

Dr. Hamby's analytical mind has been an invaluable component of his ability to classify, organize, and record surgical and clinical experiences in a most useful and meaningful fashion. Never one to be idle, he repeatedly performed yeoman service in collating and cataloging clinical and operative data.

Born in Ennis, Texas, Dr. Hamby lived most of his early life in Georgia, which probably accounts for his warm, friendly manner and for the Southern drawl that has always remained with him. In 1924, he graduated from the University of Oklahoma Medical School. His *alma mater* bestowed upon him her Distinguished Service Award in 1967. A member of many professional and nonprofessional societies, he has served as president of the American Academy of Neurological Surgery and vice president of the Harvey Cushing Society.

Because of the Clinic's compulsory retirement ruling, our honored guest left Cleveland in November 1968, for Fort Lauderdale, Florida, where he claims to have given up the practice of neurosurgery in favor of a life of ease. Characteristically, he has entered retirement with a zest for all that it involves. His golf handicap is falling gradually, and there are scarcely open spaces left on his calendar. As might be expected, Dr. Hamby has not completely stayed away from neurosurgery but manages to find time to counsel a young neurosurgeon, new to the community, on the management of intracranial aneurysms.

DONALD F. DOHN, M.D.

Paul C. Sharkey

Dr. Sharkey was born in Washington, D.C. on May 10, 1924. He lived in several Northeastern cities where his father was a hospital administrator. His family moved to Phoenix, Arizona in 1936. During World War II he was a pilot in the United States Air Force and flew B-17s.

Dr. Sharkey attended the Arizona State University after his discharge from service and he graduated with high distinction in 1949. He then attended the Baylor University College of Medicine and received his M.D. degree from that institution. He interned at the Hamot Hospital in Erie, Pennsylvania and served his residency in neurological surgery at the Baylor system in Houston. He was at the National Hospital for Nervous Disease at Queen's Square, London in 1959. Dr. Sharkey returned to Houston as an assistant professor of neurological surgery at Baylor and later he was promoted to associate professor. He continued his work at Baylor on a half-time basis and began his own private practice. He became secretary-treasurer of the Houston Neurological Society from 1960 to 1963 and was president in 1965.

Dr. Sharkey became quite active in the Congress of Neurological Surgeons and was president at the 1969 meeting in Boston. His presidential address was memorable in that it stressed close family ties and responsibilities. Dr. Sharkey became very interested in rehabilitation and helped build an outstanding spinal injury center at the Texas Institute for Research and Rehabilitation. He assisted in the development of a phrenic pacemaker. He became very active in restorative neurology working with European and American contributors. His work in this program resulted in new diagnostic techniques and useful management techniques, particularly in the areas of movement disorders and treatment of pain. He contributed a number of papers, chapters, articles, and book reviews and has been co-editor of several books.

Dr. Sharkey married Katherine Redick in 1952 and they have two daughters, Kimberly and Sandra, and two sons, Paul and Steven. The Sharkeys also have two grandsons. Dr. Sharkey and Katherine have been active members of the Grace Lutheran Church in Houston. He has served on the Church Council and has been vice president of the congregation. Dr. Sharkey's interests include travel, hunting, fishing, working on the family farm, sports, and reading natural and Civil War history.

1970

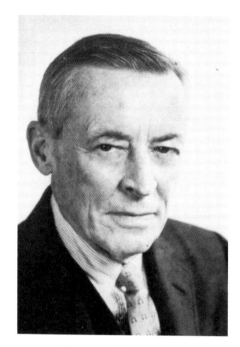

BARNES WOODHALL

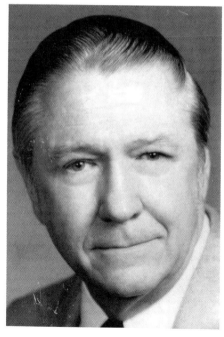

JOHN MORGAN THOMPSON

Barnes Woodhall

Barnes Woodhall was born in Rockport, Maine, on January 22, 1905. His father, Charles H. Woodhall, was one of the original executives of the Boys' Clubs of America. Because his family moved frequently while he was growing up, Dr. Woodhall received his early education at a number of schools in New England and New Jersey. He then spent his collegiate years at Williams College in Williamstown, Massachusetts, where he excelled academically and also found time to become proficient at wrestling, boxing, and ski jumping.

While he was in college, Dr. Woodhall worked during the summers in the New York offices of the American Telephone and Telegraph Company, and seemed headed toward a career as a stockbroker. Fortunately, however, his interests were diverted toward medicine in his senior year by a stimulating biology teacher. After receiving an A.B. degree from Williams College in 1926, Dr. Woodhall entered The Johns Hopkins University School of Medicine, and obtained his M.D. degree in 1930.

Even then, Dr. Woodhall showed the pioneering initiative that typified his subsequent career. On August 25, 1928, he became one of the few married medical students of that era. His bride, Frances Colman, was originally from Duluth, Minnesota. She was an excellent swimmer and was preparing for the 1924 Olympic trials when she decided instead to pursue another of her interests—medical illustration. She studied the basic illustration techniques at the Mayo Clinic and then moved to The Johns Hopkins for advanced work with Max Brödel. Among the works illustrated by Mrs. Woodhall while Dr. Woodhall was in training was *The Sign of Babinski: A Study of the Evolution of Cortical Dominance in Primates* by J. F. Fulton and A. D. Keller (Charles C Thomas, Publisher, Springfield, IL., 1932).

As a result of part-time experimental work while he was a medical student, Dr. Woodhall became interested in a career in ophthalmology. But during an internship and 7 years of surgical residency training at The Johns Hopkins, his field of interest changed. At that time, many of the basic neurosurgical techniques had been developed, but cerebral angiography, blood transfusions, antibiotics, steroids, and many other essentials of current neurosurgical practice were not yet in general use. A great deal remained to be done. After several arduous rotations on the "brain service" of Dr. Walter Dandy, Dr. Woodhall accepted the challenge of specializing in this difficult field.

When he finished his training in 1937, Dr. Woodhall was appointed to the faculty of the Duke University School of Medicine as an assistant professor with the responsibility for organizing a neurosurgical service. His first operation at Duke was a 3-hour retrogasserian neurotomy by the suboccipital approach. In his characteristically vivid operative note, he stated, "The time of this procedure was unnecessarily prolonged because of the inexperienced team, and because of the bleeding in which the operator unfortunately found himself." Also characteristically, his patient had an excellent result and recovered uneventfully.

Dr. Woodhall's initial work at Duke covered a range of neurosurgical topics, but it was interrupted by World War II. Dr. Woodhall enlisted in the Army Medical Corps in 1942, and after a stint at the Ashford General Hospital in

West Virginia, he served as chief of neurosurgery at the Walter Reed General Hospital in Washington, D.C. until 1946. During that 4-year period, Lt. Col. Woodhall helped to instruct the American general surgeons who treated the majority of acute wartime neurosurgical trauma cases, and he accumulated a broad experience in dealing with peripheral nerve injuries (for which he was awarded the Legion of Merit). Later, as a consultant to the Surgeon General and to the Veterans Administration, he served as co-editor and contributor to the two-volume history of neurosurgery in the United States Army during World War II, and as co-author of a definitive study of the peripheral nerve injuries sustained by American soldiers.

Dr. Woodhall returned to Duke University in 1946 as professor and chairman of the Division of Neurosurgery. Dr. Guy L. Odom had come to Duke in 1943, and with his help, Dr. Woodhall organized a neurosurgical residency training program there. From 1946 through 1959, 21 men entered the Duke neurosurgical residency program. Eleven remained in academic neurosurgery, and six became chairmen of their own departments.

With Dr. Odom and his various residents, Dr. Woodhall investigated a number of basic neurosurgical problems, such as peripheral nerve surgery, aneurysms and subbarachnoid hemorrhage, hypothermia, and the chemotherapy of brain tumors.

These studies, his large clinical practice, and his teaching and administrative duties filled a large portion of every day for Dr. Woodhall, but he still found time to advance neurosurgery on a national and international basis by accepting a series of editorial and organizational offices. In 1953 he became a member of the Editorial Board of the *Journal of Neurosurgery*, and he served as its chairman in 1961 and 1962. He also served on the Advisory Board of the Journal. For many years he was editor of the *American Lectures in Neurosurgery* series of monographs published by Charles C Thomas.

Dr. Woodhall was president of the American Academy of Neurological Surgeons in 1946, the Southern Neurosurgical Society in 1954, the Harvey Cushing Society from 1963 to 1964, and the Society of Neurological Surgeons from 1964 to 1965. He also served as a member of the Executive Council of the World Federation of Neurosurgical Societies in 1960 and as treasurer of the Second International Congress of Neurological Surgery, held in Washington, D.C. in 1961. In 1965 he was an honorary vice president of the Third International Congress of Neurological Surgery in Copenhagen.

While at the peak of his neurosurgical career in 1960, Dr. Woodhall began a second career as a university administrator. Dr. Odom accepted the position of chairman of the Duke Division of Neurosurgery, and Dr. Woodhall successively became dean of the Duke University School of Medicine, and assistant provost, vice provost, associate provost, and chancellor *pro tem* of Duke University. During the years from 1960 to 1969, Dr. Woodhall experienced firsthand the trials of a university executive. Largely due to his cool head and firm but understanding leadership, Duke University maintained an even keel through the turmoil of student dissent.

Dr. Woodhall's knowledge and administrative abilities also prompted his selection as an advisor or consultant to various medical groups between 1960 and 1970, such as the Health Planning Council for Central North Carolina, the National Institutes of Health, the Veterans Administration, and the American Cancer Society. From 1964 to 1968, Dr. Woodhall was a member and then chairman of the Board of Regents of the National Library of Medicine. In 1967 he journeyed to Australia to visit six universities and the Canberra Research Council to discuss the problem of the modern medical curriculum.

Despite his busy professional career, Dr. Woodhall maintained a close and harmonious family life. He and Mrs. Woodhall had the satisfaction of watching their two children mature and begin useful careers of their own, and their holidays were enlivened by visits from four grandchildren.

The years brought Dr. Woodhall additional laurels. In 1962, Dr. Woodhall's former residents gathered in Durham for a scientific and social meeting in his honor. More recently, the Duke medical alumni commissioned a portrait of Dr. Woodhall that now hangs in the Duke Hospital amphitheater. He was named James B. Duke Professor of Neurosurgery at Duke University, he was elected a Charter Member of the Society of Scholars at The Johns Hopkins University, and he was given an honorary Doctor of Science degree by Williams College. In 1965, the book *Neurosurgical Classics* was dedicated to Dr. Woodhall, and, in 1970, he was selected as the honored guest at the Annual Meeting of the Congress of Neurological Surgeons.

At the Fourth International Congress of Neurological Surgery, held in New York City in 1969, Dr. Woodhall was one of six distinguished neurosurgeons from around the world who were selected to give special lectures. Typically, Dr. Woodhall did not mention any of the areas of his previous achievements, but instead focused his attention on certain aspects of cerebral biochemical energetics, a new field that he explored with his younger colleagues. At the time when most men would be summarizing their life's work, Dr. Woodhall was looking ahead to intensified research in this exciting area. Dr. Barnes Woodhall died in March 1985.

ROBERT H. WILKINS, M.D.

John Morgan Thompson

John Morgan Thompson was born in Tampa, Florida on February 14, 1924. He attended the University of Florida and received a B.S. degree at Tulane University where he was elected to Phi Beta Kappa. He attended The Johns Hopkins School of Medicine where he worked with Dr. Clinton Woolsey in the neurophysiology laboratory during his last 3 years of medical school. He spent 6 months as a fellow in neuroanatomy at the Montreal Neurological Institute in 1946 under the direction of Dr. Wilder Penfield. He married Dorothy Georgene Kinne, a recent graduate of The Johns Hopkins School of Anesthesia, in 1947. He graduated from medical school in 1948 and was elected to Alpha Omega Alpha and Sigma Xi. He received the Borden Undergraduate Research Award in Medicine on graduation. He was a National Research Council Fellow in Neurophysiology from 1948 to 1949. He served his internship at the University of Michigan Hospital in Ann Arbor from 1949 to 1950 and then became an assistant resident in general surgery at the University of Michigan. He was called to active duty by the Navy in October 1950 and was classified as a general surgeon and was loaned to the Army. He was sent to Korea with MASH 8225 as a general surgeon and was in the forward MASH unit during 1951. He later was a general surgeon at the Corpus Christi Naval Hospital.

Dr. Thompson returned to the University of Michigan Hospital in 1952 and became an assistant resident in neurology. He then was a resident in neurological surgery under the direction of Dr. Edgar Kahn and Dr. Richard Schneider. He was invited to join the faculty of the University of Michigan when he completed his surgical residency.

Dr. Thompson has practiced neurological surgery in St. Petersburg, Florida for almost 35 years. He has been chief of staff at the All Children's Hospital and also at the Bayfront Medical Center. He has been treasurer and vice president of the Pinellas County Medical Society. Dr. Thompson has been a member of the faculty of the University of South Florida School of Medicine since it was founded 20 years ago. He has taught neuroanatomy and neurological surgery and is currently clinical professor of neurological surgery. He was invited to give the commencement address to the graduating class of the Medical School in 1977. He was a lecturer at the Stetson University School of Law from 1956 to 1980.

Dr. Thompson served on the Executive Committee of the Congress of Neurological Surgeons from 1962 to 1971. He was secretary from 1965 to 1968 and president from 1969 to 1970. He is pleased that his classmate in medical school, Dr. Walter Dandy, Jr., was able to attend the St. Louis meeting in 1970 since Dr. Walter Dandy, Sr. was born in Missouri. Dr. Thompson had the pleasure of being introduced to Dr. Walter Dandy, Sr. by his son while he was in medical school. Dr. Thompson considers it a privilege that he has had the opportunity to be associated with four of the previous honored guests of the Congress, Dr. Walter Dandy, Sr., Dr. Wilder Penfield, Dr. Edgar Kahn, and Dr. Richard Schneider.

John and Dorothy Thompson have two children. Lauralee Ann Thompson graduated from Tulane Medical School and is Board certified in both radiology and nuclear medicine. She practices in Los Angeles, California. John T. Thompson graduated from The Johns Hopkins School of Medicine and is now an associate professor at Yale Medical School where he is in charge of the retina and vitreous sections of the Department of Ophthalmology. The Thompsons have two grandchildren, one born at The Johns Hopkins and one born at Yale.

1971

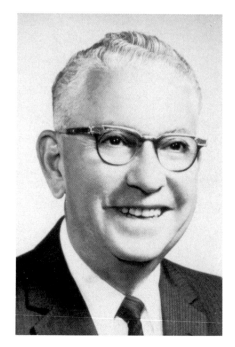

Elisha S. Gurdjian

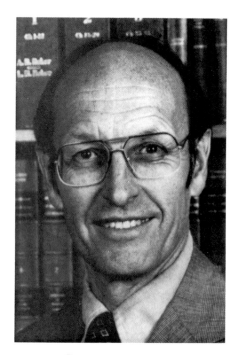

Donald F. Dohn

Elisha S. Gurdjian

In 1971, the Congress of Neurological Surgeons honored one of the giants of neurosurgery, a man who made an impact in the fields of basic research, clinical excellence, applied research, and education. Because of him and others like him, there are fewer giants in neurosurgery, for they, through their fine training programs, have elevated the stature of *all* neurosurgeons.

It is always difficult to select the most distinguished accomplishment from such a varied career, but I suspect that Dr. Gurdjian himself might choose his doctoral dissertation on "The Diencephalon of the Rat" (3), published in 1927 under the guidance of Drs. Carl G. Huber and Elizabeth C. Crosby, his advisors in the Department of Anatomy at the University of Michigan. On the other hand, I would select the basic work done in biomechanical investigation, "Mechanism of Head Injury as Studied by the Cathode Ray Oscilloscope— Preliminary Report." In conjunction with his colleague Professor Herbert Lissner, Dr. Gurdjian clearly established the practicality of combined disciplinary research associating neurosurgeons and engineers, thereby giving origin to important discipline of bioengineering. Residents are likely to remember him best as a teacher and counselor whose direct comment and embarrassing questions soon developed the trainees' areas of strength and weakness.

Dr. Gurdjian was born in Smyrna, Asia Minor, in April 1900. He attended the International College in Smyrna and graduated from there with an A.B. in 1919. He came to Michigan in 1920 and entered the University of Michigan Medical School. After the war between Greece and Turkey from 1921 to 1922, his family emigrated to Athens, Greece.

During his time in medical school Dr. Gurdjian came to the attention of Dr. Huber, chairman of the Department of Anatomy, and became involved in a combined medical and graduate program, receiving his M.S. in 1924, his M.D. in 1926, and his Ph.D. in 1927. After a period of internship and general surgical training, Dr. Gurdjian entered the residency training program of Dr. Max Peet at the University of Michigan, immediately following Dr. Edgar A. Kahn, our guest in 1964. Upon completion of his residency training program, Dr. Gurdjian moved to Detroit and began his clinical practice of neurosurgery, a practice in which he was still actively engaged in 1971.

Neurosurgery was established as a separate department in the Wayne State University School of Medicine in 1957 and Dr. Gurdjian was appointed the department's first professor and chairman, a post he held until his Medical School retirement in July 1970. In 1971, he was professor emeritus in the Department of Neurosurgery and was continuing his activities within the department, planning for changes in his textbook, *Operative Neurosurgery*, and writing a monograph about his studies in the field of impact head injury.

Although Dr. Gurdjian practiced neurosurgery in many hospitals throughout the city in his early years, he has for the most part confined his clinical activities to the Grace Hospital, of which he was chief of staff from 1961 to 1963, and to the Detroit General Hospital (formerly Receiving Hospital) where he was also chief of staff in 1952. In 1971, he was active in the clinical practice of neurosurgery, but he had turned over most of his hospital functions to his colleagues in private practice and to his successors in the department at the school.

Dr. Gurdjian and Dr. John E. Webster, his former associate, were early interested in the neurosurgical aspects of cerebrovascular disease and did much to promulgate the use of angiography in the study of this disease. The Department of Neurosurgery at Wayne under Dr. Gurdjian's direction was an active member of the cooperative study of extracranial cerebral vascular disease until that study was phased out and replaced by the randomized series. Dr. Gurdjian was likewise responsible for leading his associates and the department into the cooperative study of nontraumatic subarachnoid hemorrhage from the inception of the study to its termination.

By 1971, Dr. Gurdjian had authored alone, or in collaboration, 326 papers and publications. He was at that time, the author of two books, one of which had just completed its third edition. He was the editor of numerous compilations and symposia. He pioneered in the concept of collaborative and team research as evidenced by the multiple authors noted on many of his publications. Sixteen residents have completed their training under his direction and more than half hold academic positions, including one departmental chairmanship. In addition, three men have taken their doctorates in bioengineering under Dr. Gurdjian's direction. One of these men, Dr. Voigt R. Hodgson, remained to take charge of the Biomechanics Laboratory of the Department of Neurosurgery at Wayne State University.

Dr. Gurdjian refers to himself as primarily a neurosurgeon and not an administrator. It seems appropriate to allude to his two favorite operative procedures, i.e., trigeminal rhizotomy or decompression and cervical laminectomy. To those of us who trained under him, the ease with which he would gain access to the trigeminal nerve often seemed unbelievable.

In 1933 Dr. Gurdjian married Dorothy Eileen Kratz, his close companion of these many years. Mrs. Gurdjian has fortunately enjoyed the rapidly moving life selected by her husband with its many short trips to this meeting or that meeting. They have four children, one of whom is also a neurosurgeon presently practicing in Williamsport, Pennsylvania.

Dr. Gurdjian is a member of many learned societies, belonging to the Society of Neurological Surgeons, the American Association of Neurological Surgeons, the Congress of Neurological Surgeons, the American Neurological Association, the American College of Surgeons and is, of course, a diplomate of the American Board of Neurological Surgery. He served as a member of this Board from 1962 to 1968 and often remarked that this was one of his finest experiences. He served as a consultant for the National Institutes of Health as a member of the Special Projects Committee of the National Heart Institute from 1964 to 1967.

All who trained under his guidance must remember his exhortation that work—hard work—is the best way to solve problems, to cope with sadness or despair, and to curb excessive self-satisfaction. To many of us he was and is like a father—a stern, critical, demanding, self-centered, forgiving, helpful, lovable father. I remember the "Professor" as recently as yesterday and look forward to a host of tomorrows for his criticism, help, counsel, judicious needling, and kind understanding. His influence and counsel will continue, God willing, for years to come.

L. M. Thomas, M.D.

Donald F. Dohn

Donald F. Dohn was born on August 16, 1925 in Buffalo, New York. He attended the Kenmore public schools in Tonawanda, New York. He received his premedical education at the University of Buffalo in Buffalo, New York. He graduated from the University of Buffalo School of Medicine in 1952 and received a Baccelli Research Award and was elected to the Alpha Omega Alpha Honorary Medical Society. He was a member of the Nu Sigma Nu fraternity while in medical school. He served a rotating internship at the Buffalo General Hospital and then went to the Cleveland Clinic where he was a resident in general surgery from 1953 to 1954 and a resident in neurological surgery from 1954 to 1958. He was a clinical clerk in neurology and neuropathology (Fulbright Scholar) at the Institute of Neurology, National Hospital, Queen's Square, London from October 1956 to June 1957. He toured neurosurgical centers in Great Britain and Europe between June and August 1957 and toured neurosurgical centers in England, Sweden, France, and Switzerland in June and July 1970. He also visited the University of Vermont in Burlington, Vermont and its microsurgical laboratory. He joined the neurosurgical staff at the Cleveland Clinic in 1958 and was chairman of the Department of Neurosurgery from 1968 until 1981. He then moved to Pascagoula, Mississippi and joined the active staff of the Singing River Hospital. Dr. Dohn moved to Fort Lauderdale, Florida in January 1988 where he joined the staff of the Department of Neurosurgery at the Cleveland Clinic in Florida.

Dr. Dohn was certified by the American Board of Neurological Surgery in 1960 and became an associate examiner in 1969 and served as a member of the Board from 1972 to 1977. Dr. Dohn joined the Congress of Neurological Surgeons (CNS) in 1959 and was a member of the Executive Committee from 1965 to 1977 and was chairman of the Annual Meeting Committee in 1968. He was president of the CNS in 1971 when the meeting was held in Miami.

Dr. Dohn is a member of the American Academy of Neurological Surgeons and the American College of Surgeons. He served on the Board of Directors of the American Association of Neurological Surgeons (AANS) from 1968 to 1981 and was treasurer from 1974 to 1977. He served as president of the AANS in 1979. Dr. Dohn is a member of the Society of Neurological Surgeons, the Southern Neurosurgical Society, and the Florida Neurosurgical Society. He has published 62 papers on a wide variety of neurosurgical topics. Dr. Dohn has three children, Debra born on May 6, 1953; Douglas born on May 10, 1955; and David born on August 20, 1958. He and his wife, Carolyn, are quite fond of sailing, a sport that he has enjoyed in both Mississippi and Florida.

1972

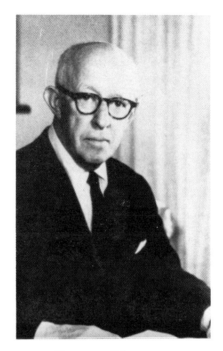

Francis Murphey

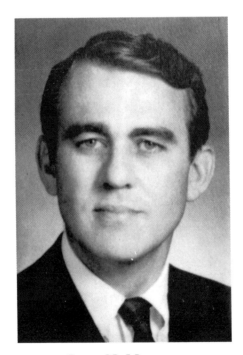

John N. Meagher

Francis Murphey

Francis Murphey was born on the 24th of December 1906, in Macon, Mississippi, the son of Edwin Mason Murphey and Clara Virginia Boggess. He attended school in Macon, and then graduated with an A.B. degree from Vanderbilt University. He received his M.D. degree from the Harvard Medical School. Dr. Murphey served a surgical internship at the University of Chicago Hospitals in Chicago, Illinois during 1933 and 1934. While he was in Chicago, Dr. Paul Bucy suggested to him the possibility of associating with Dr. Eustace Semmes in Memphis, Tennessee. Dr. Murphey joined Dr. Semmes in 1934, and completed a residency in neurological surgery at the University of Tennessee Medical Center with Dr. Semmes. Dr. Murphey sequentially held every academic rank in the Department of Neurosurgery at the University of Tennessee, culminating in his appointment as professor and chairman in 1956. In addition to his duties at the University of Tennessee, he was able to direct an active service at the Baptist Memorial Hospital and was named chief of service of the Department of Neurosurgery in 1956.

With the outbreak of World War II, Dr. Murphey entered the Armed Services. He was chief of the Neurosurgical Service at O'Reilly General Hospital in Springfield, Missouri, a center for peripheral nerve injuries, from 1942 to 1946. This offered an unusual opportunity for Dr. Murphey, and with his characteristic astuteness and energy he made the most of the opportunity, becoming a leading authority on the diagnosis and treatment of injuries of the peripheral nerves. In 1947 he became the first to demonstrate the myelographic picture of cervical nerve root avulsion. His chapter on peripheral nerve injuries that appeared in *Campbell's Operative Orthopaedics* is one of the most lucid works on this subject. Dr. Murphey still maintains an intense interest in injuries to peripheral nerves and enjoys demonstrating the clinical diagnosis of these injuries to medical students and residents.

Another disorder that attracted Dr. Murphey's attention was ruptured lumbar and cervical discs, and the subsequent work of Dr. Murphey and Dr. Semmes in this field has become legend. Dr. Murphey shared some of his experiences with the members of the Congress of Neurological Surgeons at the 1972 meeting.

Dr. Murphey has also had a particular interest in cerebrovascular problems. As director of the University of Tennessee Cerebrovascular Research Center, he contributed to the cooperative studies that have investigated subarachnoid hemorrhage and extracranial occlusive disease. He directed research on these problems for a number of years, with a special emphasis on profound hypothermia and its application toward the treatment of aneurysms and other vascular lesions of the brain.

His talents were recognized early by the many neurosurgical organizations of which he has been a member. He was president of the American Academy of Neurological Surgery in 1942, president of the Southern Neurosurgical Society in 1964, and president of the American Association of Neurological Surgeons in 1966. In addition, he has served on the American Board of Neurological Surgery and was its chairman in 1964. He was president and chief of staff of the Baptist Memorial Hospital, and was named a consultant to the National Institutes of Health in 1962.

Dr. Murphey is the author of many scientific papers and chapters in books. However, he has still found time to pursue his avid fascination with hunting, fishing, gin rummy, and golf. He approaches these with the same thoroughness that he does neurosurgery. On one occasion, he took some of his friends for breakfast in a small cafe prior to a duck hunt. When the proprietor regretted that he had no eggs to serve for their breakfast, Dr. Murphey remarked, "I thought this might happen," and produced the eggs which he had brought with him as a precaution.

Dr. Murphey has a reputation as an astute clinician and he is an extremely thorough examiner. He has a remarkable memory for unusual cases. He never makes a snap diagnosis, although it sometimes appears that he arrives at the diagnosis very quickly. His diagnosis is always based on a very careful analysis of the patient's history, physical findings, and all related information.

He is outspoken on those subjects with which he is familiar, and he is always able to back his opinions with facts. He is never afraid to take a stand, even though this stand may be unpopular, and it usually develops that the unpopular stand is the correct one.

Dr. Murphey is married to Roder Trigg of Memphis. They have one daughter, Elizabeth Coulon Murphey Ransom, and two grandchildren, Beth and Jennifer. Dr. Murphey is convinced that he is the only grandfather who will have two Miss Americas as grandchildren.

It is a privilege to have been associated with Dr. Murphey over the past 20 years. He has inspired those who have been associated with him to be thorough in their clinical approach, to be certain of their facts when they make statements, and to consider all the factors involved, whether it be treating a patient, conducting a scientific meeting, or arranging for a duck hunt.

RICHARD L. DeSAUSSURE, JR., M.D.

John N. Meagher

Dr. John N. Meagher was born on December 23, 1925 in Springfield, Ohio. He attended public schools and then entered Kenyon College. He served a 36-month tour in the United States Navy in the Aviation Division. He then returned to Kenyon College and was awarded a B.A. degree in 1946. He attended the University of Cincinnati School of Medicine and received his M.D. degree in 1950. He served his internship at the White Cross Hospital in Columbus, Ohio from 1950 to 1951 and then served residencies in neurology and neurological surgery at the same institution. He was a fellow in neurological surgery at the Barnes Hospital at Washington University, St. Louis, Missouri from 1955 to 1956 and then chief resident in neurosurgery at the Ohio State University Hospital in Columbus, Ohio from 1956 to 1957. He taught neuroanatomy for 3 years between 1951 and 1953. He was a full-time assistant professor of neurological surgery at Ohio State University from 1957 to 1959. He then entered private practice in 1959 but continued on the clinical faculty of the Ohio State University and was named clinical professor of neurological surgery in 1973. He was named professor emeritus in the Department of Surgery, Ohio State University in 1987. Dr. Meagher was certified by the American Board of Neurological Surgery in 1958. He was director of neurosurgical education at the Riverside Methodist Hospital from 1961 until he retired in 1984.

Dr. Meagher was very active in the Congress of Neurological Surgeons (CNS). He chaired a committee that was responsible for putting on the first live operative clinic in the United States. Drs. Wallace Hamby and Donald Matson were two of the noted surgeons at the live operative neurosurgical clinic in Chicago in 1965. Dr. Meagher helped expand the work of the Socio-Economic Committee and expanded the Annual Meeting to include breakfast seminars and luncheon seminars. Dr. Meagher was President of the CNS from 1971 to 1972 and served as president at the meeting in Denver. He fondly recalls how extremely well informed, cooperative, and helpful were members of his Executive Committee.

Dr. Meagher was president of the Columbus Academy of Medicine and was a delegate to the Ohio State Medical Association between 1972 and 1976. He is a past president of the Ohio State Neurosurgical Society. He was president of the Neurosurgical Society of America from 1979 to 1980 and has been vice president of the Society of Neurological Surgeons. He was on the Board of Directors of the American Association of Neurological Surgeons from 1972 to 1975 and was a member of the American Board of Neurological Surgery from 1981 to 1986. He has been a member of the Advisory Council of Neurological Surgery of the American College of Surgeons. He has served on the Board of Trustees at the Riverside Methodist Hospital from 1978–1984. Dr. Meagher has been the author of 20 publications. He was named the Ohio Neurosurgeon of the Year in 1985.

Dr. Meagher married Maxine A. Grouve on July 31, 1948. Dr. and Mrs. Meagher have three children: Michael who is 42 years of age and is a neurosurgeon; Steven, 36, who is an attorney; and John who is 26 years of age and a senior in college. Dr. Meagher had the good fortune of practicing neurological surgery with his son for 5 years prior to his retirement in March 1984.

1973

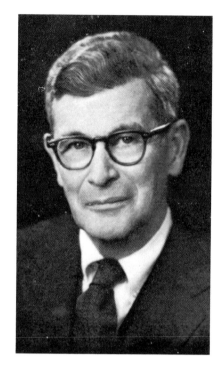

HENRY GERARD SCHWARTZ

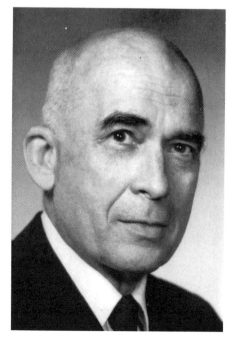

BERNARD SUTHERLAND PATRICK

Henry Gerard Schwartz

Henry Gerard Schwartz, our distinguished honored guest, was born in New York City in 1909. In 1928 he received his undergraduate degree from Princeton University, and he earned his M.D. from The Johns Hopkins University in 1932. His interest in the nervous system began during college days and, after arriving at Hopkins, acquired new momentum under the stimulating tutelage of the great neuroanatomist, Marion Hines. For the work constituting his first publication on regeneration of nervous tissue he received the Howell Award for Student Research. During the last year of medical school he spent several months in the clinic of Otfrid Foerster, a man whose remarkable character remained indelibly impressed upon him. Doubtless his greatest good fortune at Hopkins, however, was to meet and, later, to win the hand of classmate Edith Robinson, the lovely and charming Reedie who shares his honor today.

Following a general surgical internship at Hopkins he pursued his interest in anatomy as the National Research Council Fellow at Harvard Medical School for 2 years where he also served as instructor in anatomy from 1935 to 1936. To this day his interest in anatomy is reflected in a number of his scientific papers, by the precision of surgical dissection and in daily colloquy with colleagues and residents.

He began his training in neurological surgery with Dr. Ernest Sachs at Washington University School of Medicine in 1936 and served as instructor in neurological surgery from 1937 to 1942. From 1942 to 1945 he served as a member of the Washington University 21st Army Hospital in Africa and in Italy, achieving the rank of lieutenant colonel and receiving the Legion of Merit in 1945. His loyalty and devotion to maintenance of the highest standards of neurosurgical care in the military service has continued over the years in his capacity as consultant to the Surgeon General of the U.S. Army.

In 1945 Dr. Schwartz returned to St. Louis and in 1946 he was appointed professor and chairman of the Division of Neurological Surgery at Washington University, inaugurating the period of his most consuming professional interest since that time, the training of neurological surgeons and investigators. The now legendary rigors which have characterized his clinical training program, together with the opportunities afforded residents from an unusually close alliance that he has established with colleagues in neurology and the basic sciences, have provided an extraordinary milieu for attracting outstanding men to the challenge. Many have subsequently established their own training programs and have achieved distinction in neurological surgery.

Dr. Schwartz's own distinctions and contributions to neurological surgery have been numerous. His clinical interests have centered on surgery of pain, intracranial aneurysms, and pituitary and angle tumors. He designed one of the first spring vascular clips, subsequently elaborated upon by many others.

His leadership in societies and associations related to neurosurgery has continued to the present. A member of the American Academy of Neurological Surgery since 1942, he served as its vice president in 1950 and president in

1951. He also served as president of the Southern Neurosurgical Society from 1952 to 1953, the American Association of Neurological Surgeons (Harvey Cushing Society) 1967 to 1968, and the Society of Neurological Surgeons in 1968. He was installed as first vice president of the American College of Surgeons in 1972. He is a member of the American Association of Anatomists, American Surgical Association, Association for Research in Nervous and Mental Diseases, Central Neuropsychiatric Association, Deutsche Gesellschaft fur Neurochirurgie, Excelsior Surgical Society, Alpha Omega Alpha, Sigma Xi, Societe Internationale de Chirurgie, Societa Italiana di Neurochirurgia, Societe de Neurochirurgie de Langue Francaise, and Society of Medical Consultants to the Armed Forces. In 1962 he served as visiting professor at the Free University of West Berlin.

He served on the Editorial Board of the *Journal of Neurosurgery* from 1958 to 1967, and as chairman in 1968. He worked as a member of the American Board of Neurological Surgery from 1964 to 1970, serving as chairman from 1968 to 1970, and received their Distinguished Service Award in 1970.

Over the years, he has willingly accepted many special committee responsibilities with national societies and governmental agencies, reflecting his concern for academic excellence and postgraduate training. He was a member of the Advisory Council for Neurological Surgery, American College of Surgeons (1949–1952 and 1960–1965, chairman, 1965); regional representative, The Johns Hopkins Medical School Committee on Admissions; member of the Neurology Study Section, National Institutes of Health (1958–1962); member of the Neurology Training Grant Committee, National Institutes of Health (1956–1960); delegate, World Federation of Neurosurgical Societies; and member of the Graduate Training Committee, American College of Surgeons (1960–1965); Peripheral Nerve Subcommittee, American Medical Association (1961–1963); Ladue Board of Education (1955–1960); Board of Scientific Counselors, National Institute of Neurological Diseases and Blindness, National Institutes of Health (1964–1968); Joint Committee for Stroke Facilities; and the American Surgical Association, American College of Surgeons Committee to Study Surgical Services for the United States.

Despite these time-consuming responsibilities, he served as acting head of the Department of Surgery of Washington University School of Medicine from 1965 through 1967, and in 1970 was named the August A. Busch Jr. Professor of Neurological Surgery. His outstanding contributions to Washington University were recognized in 1969 by the Alumni Federation Faculty Award.

When free of these endeavors, he most enjoys the congenial company of his three sons and his grandchildren, a fast set of tennis, peering from a duck blind on crisp Missouri mornings, or searching for the ideal stream in which to cast a dry fly. To his many friends, colleagues, associates, and residents, past and present, Henry Schwartz emerges a man of extraordinary character, vigor, and integrity, a consummate clinician and surgeon, compassionate physician to the sick, rigorous teacher, valuable and willing counselor, and one possessed of unswerving loyalty to person, country, and his own ideals.

WILLIAM S. COXE, M.D.

Bernard Sutherland Patrick

Bernard Sutherland Patrick was born in Booneville, Mississippi, February 16, 1927. He grew up in Corinth, Mississippi and was a fourth generation physician in his family. His undergraduate studies were at Tulane University and the University of Mississippi. He graduated from the University of Illinois in Chicago in 1950 with his M.D. degree. At Illinois he was elected to Pi Kappa Epsilon, a scholastic honorary fraternity. Dr. Patrick interned at Augustana Hospital in Chicago and was influenced by neurosurgeon Wesley Axel Gustafson. This association led Dr. Patrick toward neurosurgery. Dr. Patrick served 2 years as a flight surgeon during the Korean War but returned to Chicago to train under Eric Oldberg at the Illinois Neuropsychiatric Institute of the University of Illinois. Dr. Patrick was invited by Drs. Semmes and Murphey of Memphis to develop the neurosurgical laboratory at the University of Tennessee in 1957. Because of lack of funding, the laboratory development was delayed so he entered into private practice with Drs. Semmes and Murphey in 1957. Dr. Patrick became a diplomate of the American Board of Neurological Surgery in 1960. In 1968 he was invited to join the faculty at the University of Mississippi. He moved to Jackson, Mississippi and was active in teaching and research for 10 years. He has published 14 papers with interests primarily in discography, pain management and therapy of glioblastoma. Dr. Patrick introduced anterior cervical interbody fusion and lumbar discography in the mid-South area while in Memphis.

From 1972 to 1973 Dr. Patrick became president of the Congress of Neurological Surgeons after serving 3 years as secretary. It was mainly through his efforts that the Congress of Neurological Surgeons developed its current monthly journal, *Neurosurgery*. While Dr. Patrick was president-elect of the Congress, he developed plans for a new neurosurgical journal founded by the Congress. Before these plans could be brought to fruition, Dr. Paul Bucy resigned as editor of the *Journal of Neurosurgery* and announced a new publication, *Surgical Neurology* with Dr. Bucy as publisher and editor. Conversations between Drs. Bucy and Patrick resulted in a proposal by Dr. Bucy that the Congress designate *Surgical Neurology* as its official publication. After much debate the Executive Committee felt this would be better than publishing what would be a third neurosurgical journal. Thus, the Congress announced *Surgical Neurology* as its official publication and joined in a tentative agreement with Dr. Bucy pending resolution of a firm long-term contract. Drs. Patrick, Albert Rhoton, Robert Wilkins, and Bruce Sorenson were charged with the task of negotiating the final contract with Dr. Bucy. Despite everyone's efforts to negotiate in good faith, the talks ended in a stand-off and the Congress severed its ties to *Surgical Neurology*.

Dr. Patrick belongs to the Society of Neurological Surgeons, the American Association of Neurological Surgeons, the Southern Neurosurgical Society, and the American College of Surgeons. In 1950 he married Jo Irene Kurns of Chicago, Illinois. They have four daughters, Karen, Kimberly, Kristen, and Kathleen. Since resuming private practice in Jackson, Mississippi in 1978, Dr. Patrick has devoted more time to nonmedical activities. He plays a clarinet in a woodwind quintet that rehearses twice a month at his home and has actively pursued tennis. In 1987, he and his wife won the mixed-doubles competition at the World Medical Tennis Association in Sweden playing against 42 teams from 15 countries. Dr. Patrick also flies an open-cockpit biplane and does smoke-writing in the sky.

1974

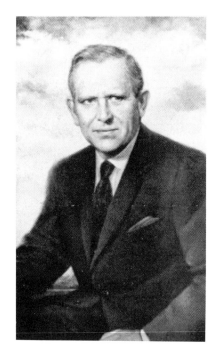

Guy L. Odom

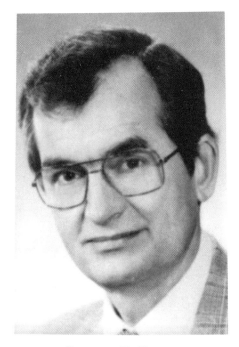

George T. Tindall

Guy L. Odom

Judging by the number of times his advice is sought each day by his residents, his associates at the Duke University Medical Center, and by numerous neurosurgeons practicing in other areas, it is readily apparent that Guy L. Odom, M.D., is, and has been for many years, a neurosurgeon's neurosurgeon. But from the number and variety of other individuals who consult, telephone, or visit him, it is also apparent that he is much more—a physician in the Hippocratic tradition, and an intuitive human being with a genuine concern for others and a zest for living.

Dr. Odom's main consideration is the welfare of his patients. He loves the clinical practice of neurosurgery, devoting as much of his energy as possible to it. In addition, he enjoys sharing this consuming interest with others in his highly successful role as teacher and residency program director. An accomplished neuropathologist, Dr. Odom has also had some interest in experimental neurosurgery as well, but he prefers the daily realities of a patient-oriented practice to the more hypothetical considerations of purely scientific research. Likewise, he is impatient with his administrative chores, which detain him from his patients, and over the years he has discharged his many national responsibilities primarily from a sense of duty.

A man with unyielding views of right and wrong, and of proper medical ethics and etiquette, Dr. Odom demonstrates well in his daily activities the correct way to conduct a neurosurgical practice. He places a premium on personal integrity and honesty, demanding it in his residents and associates. He stands by his word, and expects others to do the same. Heaven help them if they don't!

It would be an understatement to say simply that Guy Odom is not a spineless man. With his commonsense approach to life and to the practice of neurosurgery, he has always been on sure footing. Little escapes his detection, and he is not a man to let a sleeping dog lie. If he thinks that one of his residents has shown a hint of laziness, that one of his peers has let the quality of his residency program slip a little, or that a governmental agency is beginning to infringe on neurosurgeons' affairs, he reacts immediately and directly. Never one to avoid a confrontation, Dr. Odom speaks directly, in language that leaves little doubt about his meaning, and he seldom comes away second best.

Yet Guy Odom abhors publicity. In his role as one of the major leaders of American neurosurgery, he prefers to accomplish his work behind the scenes. He is embarrassed by persons or events that call attention to his achievements, such as the present biographical sketch, and for this reason I won't dwell further on the many traits and qualities that have endeared him to so many. Let us instead find out how Dr. Odom came to be the type of man he is.

In 1904, Guy Leroy Odom came to New Orleans from Plant City, Florida, to attend Tulane Medical School; there he met and married Marion Brown. Shortly thereafter, Guy's brother, Marvin, who already had an M.D. degree from Emory University, also moved to New Orleans. As fate would have it, he met and married Marion's sister, Yetta Brown. The two brothers established separate general practices and in 1915, Guy Odom became coroner of Jefferson Parish.

Two boys, Charles and Guy Leary, and a girl, Vada, were born to Guy and Marion Odom before Dr. Odom's untimely death of influenza in 1918. At that time, Charles Odom was 9 years old and Guy was 7. Their uncle watched over the family, but they were maintained largely by their own determination and ingenuity. Marion Odom, and later Charles Odom, both became pharmacists. They ran a drug store in the same small building in Harvey, Louisiana, in which Dr. Marvin Odom had his office. Thus, Guy Leary Odom grew up in a medical atmosphere, helping his mother and brother in their pharmacy and his uncle in his medical practice.

The two boys became somewhat interested in surgery during the years they served as dieners for their uncle, who had followed their father as coroner. But the event that sealed their fate occurred in 1923, when Charlie was 14 and Guy was 12—the two boys successfully amputated the leg of their injured collie under chloroform anesthesia, and subsequently fashioned him an artificial limb.

Charles preceded Guy at McDonogh-Jefferson High School, Tulane University, and Tulane Medical School, where he exhibited exceptional ability. He trained in general surgery at Charity Hospital in New Orleans, and subsequently has had an outstanding career as a general surgeon, not only in civilian life, but also as General George S. Patton's personal physician during World War II. Incidentally, Charles also succeeded his uncle as coroner of Jefferson Parish.

Guy has always looked up to his brother, and it was natural that he should follow in his footsteps. He completed undergraduate school in two full years, and was graduated from Tulane Medical School in 1933 at the age of 21. But he did not follow Charles into general surgery.

During his years as a medical student, Guy had developed an interest in the nervous system, largely due to the influence of Dr. Sidney Bliss, professor of biochemistry. Only one man was performing operations on the nervous system in New Orleans at that time, and after watching him operate, Dr. Odom decided that neurosurgery was a field to which he might contribute. After investigating the opportunities for training, Dr. Odom made up his mind to apply for a position at the Montreal Neurological Institute, due to be opened in 1934. However, the residency paid little besides room and board, and he was engaged to be married to Suzanne Price from San Antonio in August. So he accepted an interim position at the East Louisiana State Hospital, where he served for 4 years.

Then Guy and Suzanne Odom spent the years from 1937 to 1942 in Montreal, where Dr. Odom came to know two men who strongly influenced his neurosurgical development. Dr. Wilder Penfield gave him a broad outlook on the neurological sciences, and showed him the advantages of an academic practice and a close family life. Dr. William V. Cone taught him by example the importance of round-the-clock, nit-picking attention to the details of patient care and surgical technique, as well as the value of sound surgical judgment. Dr. Odom advanced through the 5-year pyramid, rotating through experimental neurosurgery, neurology, clinical neurosurgery, and neuropathology before becoming resident in neurosurgery from 1941 to 1942.

The Odoms returned to New Orleans in 1942. Dr. Odom tried to enlist in the Army, but was rejected for medical reasons, so he began a neurosurgical practice. Soon he was seeing patients at a number of hospitals, spending much of his day in transit between them. Most of these hospitals were not equipped for neurosurgical operations, and conditions were difficult. The prevailing attitude was that neurosurgical patients were not expected to recover, and that time and money spent in their behalf was wasted. Even at Charity Hospital, where his brother Charles was director, neurosurgical instruments were not purchased until after Dr. Odom had performed a dramatically successful 11th-hour trephination for a brain abscess with makeshift equipment. Dr. Odom was appointed instructor in neurosurgery at Louisiana State University and looked forward to academic advancement in the ensuing years.

However, in 1943 he was contacted by a very persistent man, Dr. Deryl Hart, professor of surgery at Duke University, who finally persuaded him to come to Durham, North Carolina, for a look. Dr. Odom accepted a position as associate in neurosurgery and has remained at the Duke University Medical Center since that time, rising through the academic ranks to become professor in 1950, chairman of the Division of Neurosurgery in 1960, and James B. Duke Professor of Neurological Surgery in 1974.

Dr. Odom has especially enjoyed having his patients' beds under the same roof as his office, examining rooms, operating rooms, and laboratories. Not only has this arrangement minimized the time he has spent getting from one to the other, but it has facilitated unification of the Division of Neurosurgery at Duke, where five staff neurosurgeons and the resident staff round together daily on the combined patients of all, and are frequently called to the operating room to consult on each other's cases.

Dr. Barnes Woodhall, honored guest of the Congress of Neurological Surgeons in 1970 (1), was away in the Army when Dr. Odom arrived in Durham in 1943, but he returned in 1946. The two men, with different backgrounds and different temperaments, found themselves associated, neither one having selected the other. Yet because of their respect for each other and their similar demand for excellence, they found to their pleasure that they got along very well together. Dr. Odom became certified by the American Board of Neurological Surgery in 1946, and in that same year the two men began a neurosurgical residency program. From then until 1974, 35 men have finished the Duke program; most spent 5 years in rotations similar to those that Dr. Odom went through at the Montreal Neurological Institute, but without the pyramid system. Fifteen of these men have taken academic positions, and in 1974, seven had become professors.

Dr. Odom's bibliography bears witness to his productivity since 1946. It is especially impressive when one considers that Dr. Odom has expended his major effort on his tremendous clinical practice and on the instruction of "his boys," rather than on experimental investigations.

On the national scene, Dr. Odom has also accomplished a great deal despite two personal setbacks—a serious coronary occlusion in 1960 and the death of his wife, Suzanne, in 1965. He has been vice president (1951) and president (1967) of the Southern Neurosurgical Society, president (1967) of the American Academy of Neurological Surgery, secretary-treasurer (1960–1965) and president (1970–1971) of the Society of Neurosurgical Surgeons, and president

(1971–1972) of the American Association of Neurological Surgeons. In addition, he has been member (1962–1964), secretary-treasurer (1964–1970), and president (1970–1972) of the American Board of Neurological Surgery; member (1964–1972) of the American Board of Medical Specialties, member (1964–1970) and chairman (1970–1972) of the Residency Review Committee for Neurological Surgery; chairman (1970–1971) of the Joint Council Subcommittee on Cerebrovascular Disease of the National Heart and Lung Institute, and the National Institute of Neurological Diseases and Stroke; Member (1968–1971) of the National Advisory Neurological Diseases and Stroke Council of the National Institutes of Health; and a member of, or consultant to, many other national, regional, and local medical groups. In 1968, Dr. Odom and Dr. C. Hunter Shelden visited 20 British neurosurgical training centers for the American Board of Neurological Surgery to assess the possibilities of establishing resident exchanges.

One would think from this list that Dr. Odom would have had to desert his own patients and residents to fulfill his national obligations. On the contrary, with thoughtful timing of trips, skillful juggling of airline arrangements, and frequent telephone calls back to Durham, Dr. Odom has been able to minimize his absences. This has been just as well, from his residents' standpoint, because these trips have always been followed by a transient surge of activity, with an increase in Dr. Odom's already over-loaded schedule.

Dr. Odom has been honored by the Neurosurgeon Award of the American Academy of Neurological Surgery (1972) and the Distinguished Service Award of the American Board of Neurological Surgery (1972) and by his selection as the Semmes Lecturer of the Southern Neurosurgical Society (1974). In 1964, his residents met in Durham to pay him tribute; in 1972 the former Duke residents met again to form the Odom-Woodhall Legion, adopting the owl as the emblem of the group, and planning meetings every 2 or 3 years. In 1973, the book, *Neurological Classics* (2), was dedicated to him.

By his example, Dr. Odom has taught his residents concern not only for their patients but for their colleagues, assistants, and families as well. Much of what he has written has been designed to be of help to general practitioners of medicine, the hard-working individuals that he has admired from the time of his boyhood. He has taught some of the sons and daughters of the Durham medical community, and in turn, his son Guy Leary Odom, Jr., M.D., was taught by some of the members of these same medical families during his years as a student at the Duke University School of Medicine. In addition, Dr. Odom's home has always been a home-away-from-home for the sons and daughters of colleagues and friends attending Duke as undergraduates. As an index of the loyalty that his personality has evoked in others, Dr. Odom's secretary, Miss Beth Toms, and his laboratory technician, Mrs. Helen Johns, have each been with him since 1945.

Throughout his professional life, Dr. Odom has continued to maintain unusually close family ties. When his children were growing up, he purposely did not take up golf or other activities that might distract him from his family when he was home from the hospital. However, he has always enjoyed deep sea fishing, and many of his vacations have been spent with his brother and his sister, Mrs. Vada Reynolds, in New Orleans; these yearly fishing excursions with Charlie have continued in spite of a series of near-catastrophies in the Gulf of Mexico. In 1974, his son Guy, a general surgeon, lived with his wife Barbara and their two children in Rutherfordton, North Carolina. His daughter, Linda, a former nurse, is married to Dr. Wesley A. Cook, a staff neurosurgeon at Duke, and they and their three children live near Durham. His daughter, Carolyn, is married to a naval architect, Terry Little; they and their three children lived in Corpus Christi, Texas. Dr. Odom married Mataline Nye Council in 1967, adding her three children and now her five grandchildren to his close family circle.

In recent years, Mataline and Guy Odom have come to enjoy a brief respite each evening from their hectic activities, relaxing in their beautiful family room. At these times, Dr. Odom, usually working on a needlepoint or macrame design, seems anything but the forceful leader he is. And then comes the succession of telephone calls. . . .

ROBERT H. WILKINS, M.D.

REFERENCES

1. Wilkins, R. H. Barnes Woodhall, M.D.: A biographical sketch. Clin. Neurosurg., 18: xvii-xx, 1971.
2. Wilkins, R. H., and Brody, I.A. Neurological Classics, 204 pp. Johnson Reprint Corporation, New York, 1973.

George T. Tindall

George T. Tindall has made significant contributions to American neurosurgery. He is well respected for his surgical skills, research, publications, and leadership in neurosurgical organizations. His name is synonymous with pituitary surgery. His career has spanned several institutions; Hopkins, Duke, Galveston, and Emory. At each, Dr. Tindall honed his skills as a hard-working and exacting surgeon, teacher, researcher, and leader in the wider reaches of American neurosurgery.

Dr. Tindall was born on March 13, 1928 in Magee, Mississippi, a small town in a highly rural setting. He was active in athletics in high school, and went to college at the University of Mississippi where he graduated in 1948. He was elected to Phi Eta Sigma, an honorary scholastic society. He married Katy Hopson and they had four children during 22 years of marriage.

Dr. Tindall entered The Johns Hopkins Medical School in 1948, finishing in 1952 and graduated Alpha Omega Alpha. During that period of time he spent a clerkship of 2 months at the Peter Bent Brigham Hospital in Boston, an experience with a good deal of influence on his life. He went into the Halsted program in general surgery at The Johns Hopkins where he spent 1 year. During this time he became acquainted with Dr. Frank Otenasek, one of Dr. Dandy's former residents, who had a profound influence on his decision to enter neurosurgery. After an interim of 2 years spent as a flight surgeon in the Air Force, Dr. Tindall entered the neurosurgical training program at Duke in 1955. He spent the next 13 years at Duke. He was in residency for 6 years and on the staff for 7 years. In 1968 he was chosen to head the Department of Neurosurgery at the University of Texas Medical Branch at Galveston. In 1973, he came to Emory and under his leadership, neurosurgery at Emory has reached national and international prominence. In 1971, after the death of his wife, Katy, he married a first-year neurology resident, Dr. Suzie Cunningham, who has been wife, companion, and neurosurgical partner since.

Dr. Tindall's clinical interests have been in aneurysms, head injuries, and pituitary surgery. In addition, he had the pleasure of training his wife in neurosurgery. She has become a strong factor in neurosurgery in this country and an effective member of the faculty of Emory University School of Medicine. Dr. Tindall has been associated with many outstanding individuals in his medical career who have had a profound influence on him. These include Jack Guyton, an ophthalmologist; David Sabiston, one of his closest friends and professor of surgery at Duke; as well as Dr. Barnes Woodhall and Dr. Guy Odom, who were his teachers in neurosurgery at Duke.

Dr. Tindall has played a major role in neurosurgical organizations. He was president of the Congress of Neurological Surgeons in 1974. During his term he was a part of the negotiations with Dr. Paul Bucy to make *Surgical Neurology* the "official" journal of the Congress. The annual meeting during Dr. Tindall's presidency was in Vancouver, and Dr. Guy Odom was the honored guest. In 1989, Dr. Tindall completed his term as president of the American Association of Neurological Surgeons (AANS). There have been only seven neurosurgeons who have achieved presidency of both the Congress and the AANS. Dr. Tindall has also been president of the Georgia Neurosurgical Society, the Society of University Neurosurgeons, and the Southern Neurosurgical Society. Dr. Tindall recently completed his 6-year term as a member of the American Board of Neurological Surgery. He has a major interest in gardening and has a farm and tree nursery, which he has built into a strong business. Dr. Tindall founded the popular biweekly publication, *Contemporary Neurosurgery* and 2 years ago, Dr. Tindall launched another biweekly, *Neurosurgical Consultations*. He has coauthored two textbooks on the pituitary, *Clinical Management of Pituitary Disorders* and *Disorders of the Pituitary*.

1975

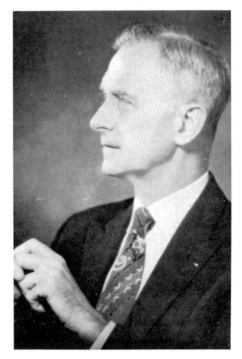

WILLIAM HERBERT SWEET

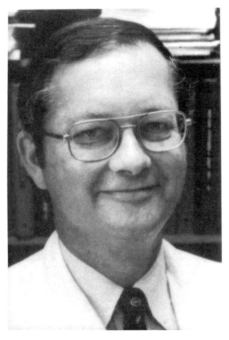

JAMES T. ROBERTSON

William Herbert Sweet

William Herbert Sweet was born on February 13, 1910 in Kerriston, Washington, the center of the timber industry in the foothills of Mount Ranier. It was soon apparent to his father, a surgeon, and his mother, a university graduate, that their first child possessed an exceptional mind. He did the first four grades in 2 years and graduated from high school at the age of 14. During this time it was also evident that he was a gifted musician and after graduation from high school he spent a year studying piano. Realizing that he did not wish to devote his life to becoming a concert artist, and undecided about his future, he worked for a year in a sawmill in Centralia, Washington.

At this point he entered the University of Washington and in 1930 graduated *summa cum laude*, first in a class of 1,000 graduates. With this brilliant academic record, he was accepted into Harvard Medical School in 1930. During his second year, he received a Rhodes Scholarship and the years of 1932 to 1934 were spent at Oxford University (Magdalen College) where he did research work in neurophysiology in the department of Sir Charles Sherrington. He received his B.Sc. degree from Oxford in 1934. On the basis of subsequent research work and publications, he was awarded a D.Sc. degree from Oxford University in 1957.

Not one to waste time or remain idle for even a short period, he utilized the Oxford vacation periods to study at the University of Würzburg (Germany) Medical School. In 1934 he took (in German) and passed the German Government Written and Oral Examinations in internal medicine. He then returned to Harvard Medical School and graduated *cum laude* with the class of 1936.

Training in neurosurgery began at the Massachusetts General Hospital in 1936 and then was continued for the next 3 years at the University of Chicago Clinic and Billings Hospital under Dr. Percival Bailey. Upon completion of his resident training in 1940, he returned to Harvard Medical School and the Massachusetts General Hospital as a Commonwealth Fund Fellow in research and for further special training in neurosurgery, especially of the autonomic nervous system.

In the early years of World War II and long before the United States' entry into that war, he actively sought a means to make explicit both his appreciation of his Rhodes scholarship and his concern over the threat to the world implicit in Hitler's Germany. This opportunity came in mid-1941 when he was asked to return to England to be the acting chief of the Queen Elizabeth Hospital, Birmingham and regional consultant in Neurosurgery to the British Emergency Medical Service in the Midlands. He served in these capacities until June 1945, and in recognition of his efforts, he later received His Majesty's Medal for Service in the Cause of Freedom. Returning to the Massachusetts General Hospital in 1945, he resumed his career in academic neurosurgery.

Early in the 1950s, Dr. Sweet, with the support of Dr. J. C. White, head of the neurosurgical service at that time and a former honored guest of the Congress, determined that advancement in knowledge in clinical neurosurgery would be accelerated if the neurosurgical service included a group of basic science investigators. To this end, Dr. Sweet established laboratories in the department of neurosurgery to include biophysics, neurophysiology, electromicroscopy, neurochemistry, and immunology with full-time members devoting their efforts to basic problems in the neurosurgical field. He was one of the first individuals to emphasize the importance of research training as part of the residency program.

In 1961 Dr. Sweet became chief of the neurosurgical service of the Massachusetts General Hospital and at the present time also holds the appointment of professor of surgery at Harvard Medical School.

His contributions to basic and clinical neurosurgery are numerous and wide ranging. His major areas of interest have included basic studies of the flow and formation of cerebrospinal fluid in man, application of radioactive isotopes to the investigation and treatment of central nervous system disorders, improvements in the techniques of clinical neurosurgery, treatment of extracranial and intracranial vascular disorders, treatment of pain, experimental investigations with primary malignant brain tumors, treatment of aggressive behavior disorders associated with organic brain disease, and medicolegal problems of neurosurgery.

In 1951 he established, with the help of his biophysical colleagues, one of the first brain scan research laboratories and the first such laboratory to be utilized routinely for clinical diagnosis. The use of coincidence counting of the annihilation radiation from positron-emitting isotopes for clinical localization of focal brain lesions was first brought to fruition there. With Dr. James C. White, he has published two classic texts on the neurosurgical treatment of pain.

He has been active in many other scientific endeavors which includes service on councils and committee study sections for the National Institute of Health, membership on the Science and Technology Advisory Committee in the office of Manned Space Flight, scientific trustee from Harvard of Associated Universities, Inc., and an editor of *Neurochirgia* and the series of volumes entitled *Progress in Neurological Surgery*. He was founding member of the Neurosciences Research Program and has been an active associate of the program since its inception. He is an honorary member of the leading neurosurgical societies of Great Britain, Spain and Portugal, Egypt, France, and a corresponding foreign member of Swiss, Italian, and Scandinavian neurosurgical societies, and a Fellow of the Royal Society of Medicine of England. He is a diplomate of both the American Board of Neurological Surgery and the American Board of Psychiatry and Neurology. Membership is also held in the American Academy of Neurology, American College of Surgeons, American Academy of Arts and Sciences, Biological Sciences (vice president, 1964–1967), American Academy of Neurological Surgery, American Association of Neurological Surgeons, American Neurological Association (vice president, 1971–1972), American Society of Stereotactic Surgery, American Physiologic Society, American Surgical Association, American Medical Association, Association for Research in Nervous and Mental Diseases, Research Society of Neurological Surgeons, Society for Neuroscience, Society of Neurological Surgeons (president, 1969–1970), Electroencephalographic Society, Boylston Medical Society, Alsted Society, New England Neurosurgical Society (president, 1957–1958), Massachusetts Medical Society, and Boston Society of Psychiatry and Neurology (president, 1957–1958).

Possessing a brilliant mind, superb technical skill, and a meticulous approach to problems in the operating room, he has supplied seemingly boundless energy to a vast number of important endeavors. Neurosurgery has been fortunate in having such an individual in its ranks for 4 decades.

ROBERT G. OJEMANN, M.D.

James T. Robertson

James T. Robertson was born April 5, 1931 in McComb, Mississippi. He is married to Valeria Brower Robertson and they have six children and four grandchildren. The youngest son, Dan, is in neurosurgical training with Dr. Grossman in Houston. The other children are business men, teachers, and secretaries.

Jim graduated from the University of Tennessee College of Medicine in December 1954 and subsequently completed his internship and neurosurgical residency in Memphis under the auspices of Eustace Semmes and Francis Murphey, completing training in 1959. He subsequently took an additional year at the Peter Bent Brigham Children's Hospital in Boston under the sponsorship of Donald Matson. He then entered the United States Medical Corps, serving as chief of neurosurgery at Travis Air Force Base, California for 3 years, and at Lackland Air Force Base Hospital as assistant chief of neurosurgery. He was discharged on June 1, 1964, with the rank of major.

Dr. Robertson returned to Memphis to practice with the Semmes-Murphey Clinic and presently is a senior partner. After demonstrating an intense interest in academic neurosurgery, he became professor and chairman of the Department of Neurosurgery at the University of Tennessee, Memphis in October 1973. He has trained more than 50 neurosurgeons.

Dr. Robertson completed the American Board of Neurological Surgery certification in October 1962. After serving on the Executive Committee of the Congress, he became president of the Congress in 1975. He has been an officer and president of the American Academy of Neurological Surgery, the Society of University Neurosurgeons, vice chairman of the Society of Neurosurgeons, and is current president of the American Association of Neurological Surgeons. He is vice chairman of the Stroke Council of the American Heart Association and a former member of the Board of Governors of the American College of Surgeons and a Delegate to the American Medical Association for the Congress of Neurological Surgeons. He has been chairman of the Joint Cerebral Vascular Section of the American Association of Neurological Surgeons and the Congress.

He has served on the Residency Review Committee for Neurological Surgery and is presently the chairman of that committee. He served as a member of the Advisory Council of the National Institute of Neurological Diseases and Stroke from 1984 to 1988. He received the Distinguished Alumni Award from the University of Tennessee, Memphis in 1990. He is a professor of anatomy and neurobiology and acting chairman of neurology at the University of Tennessee, Memphis.

He joined the PRIMUS unit of the University of Tennessee in the United States Navy Reserve in 1986 and was promoted to captain in May 1990. He recently served on active duty for 2 months at Bethesda Naval Hospital during the Persian Gulf War.

Dr. Robertson's surgical and research interests include pituitary tumors, acoustic tumors, glomus tumors, occlusive stroke, and trauma. He has served as visiting professor at a number of medical centers and his bibliography includes more than 100 articles and several book chapters.

1976

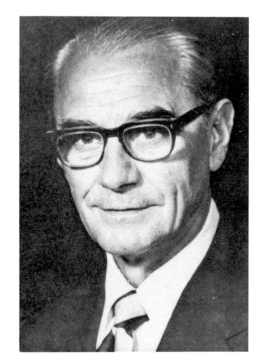

LYLE A. FRENCH

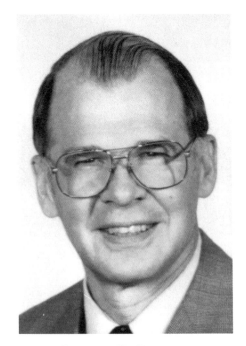

ROBERT G. OJEMANN

Lyle A. French

Lyle A. French was born in Worthing, South Dakota, March 26, 1915. His early years were spent in Lennox and Watertown, South Dakota. His family then moved to Mankato, Minnesota, where he graduated from high school. He attended Macalester College in St. Paul, where he obtained his premedical education. He then entered the University of Minnesota, where he received his B.S., M.B., and M.D. degrees, the latter being bestowed in 1940. He received his training in neurological surgery at the University of Minnesota under the guidance of Dr. William T. Peyton. Following an interruption by military service in the North African and European theatres during World War II, he completed his training in 1947, at which time he was also awarded M.S. and Ph.D. degrees in neurological surgery.

After completion of his formal training in neurosurgery, Dr. French was appointed to the neurosurgical faculty of the University of Minnesota. In 1952, he was promoted to associate professor, and in 1957 to professor. Under his guidance the Division of Neurological Surgery achieved departmental status, and he served as chairman of the department until 1974.

In recognition of his administrative capabilities, Dr. French was elected chief of staff, University Hospitals and served from 1968 to 1970. In 1970 he was appointed vice president for health science affairs at the University of Minnesota, a position which he currently holds.

Dr. French is a member of the Society of Neurological Surgeons. He served as president of the Neurosurgical Society of America in 1957 to 1958, president of the American Academy of Neurological Surgery in 1972 to 1973, and president of the American Association of Neurological Surgeons in 1973 to 1974. He was consultant to the Surgeon General, United States Army, 1963 to 1975, and was appointed consultant in neurosurgery to the Veterans Administration in 1968. He was a member of the American Board of Neurological Surgery from 1962 to 1968 and served on the Board of Editors of the *Journal of Neurosurgery* from 1970 to 1975. He was chairman of the Board of Editors of the *Journal of Neurosurgery* from 1973 to 1975. He has been a member of the Advisory Council, National Institutes of Health, National Institute of Neurological Diseases and Stroke, since 1971. Dr. French is currently a member of the Board of Governors of the American College of Surgeons. He is on the Board of Editors of the *Yearbook of Cancer* and is a member of numerous other national and international organizations.

Under his leadership as vice president for health science affairs at the University, the health sciences have undergone a steady and extensive growth and building program. This growth and development of the health sciences reflects, among other administrative attributes, Dr. French's effectiveness and capabilities in dealing with the state legislature and the federal bureaucracy.

Though his accomplishments as vice president for health science affairs have been prodigious, Dr. French is best characterized as a master neurosurgeon and as an outstanding and dedicated teacher.

His interest in teaching has encompassed all levels. He has always found it most important to bring neurosurgery to the undergraduate, as demonstrated by his personal attention to student lectures and contact on ward rounds.

At the graduate level, Dr. French created an atmosphere of creativity and curiosity. He has an incomparable capacity to bring out the best in his residents and colleagues. Above all he provided them with the opportunity and encouragement to employ their creativity and pursue their ideas. It is understandable then that Dr. French was involved in the early development of radionuclear isotope encephalometry, ultrasonic brain scanning, fundamental studies on the ultrastructure of cerebral edema, and the effects of steroids on brain edema.

As a surgeon Dr. French is a master technician. This is well established in the minds of colleagues and residents who have worked closely with him. He has contributed many published experiences on the surgical management of intracranial vascular lesions, brain tumors, pain, and seizure disorders. He also participated in the early development of endocrine ablative surgery in the management of breast cancer. He was quick to see the importance of stereotaxis in neurosurgery, and early on instituted such a program at the University Hospitals. He was elected vice president of the International Society of Stereoencephalotomy in 1967.

In 1941, Gene Richmond and Lyle French were married. Gene was originally from Paris, Missouri, and was a graduate of the University of Missouri at Columbia. Gene is a most charming lady and a devoted wife. She has always been at Lyle's side and has shared equally in the frustrations and rewards of the Professor. She has provided much support and encouragement to him. Gene and Lyle have three children, Fred, Eldridge, and Barbara, who carry with them the same warm and friendly traits as their mother and father. Fond and nostalgic memories remain in the minds of residents, colleagues, friends, and guests who have visited in the home of the French family.

As a college student, Dr. French was an outstanding athlete excelling in basketball and golf. He remains a superb golfer and enjoys hunting and fishing with many of his friends and colleagues.

It was a great privilege for the Congress of Neurological Surgeons to have Dr. Lyle A. French, a master neurosurgeon, an outstanding teacher, and a highly skilled administrator, as the honored guest at its 26th annual meeting in October 1976.

JIM L. STORY, M.D.

Robert G. Ojemann

Dr. Robert G. Ojemann was born in Iowa City, Iowa on May 5, 1931. He graduated from the University of Iowa with highest distinction and from its medical school in 1955 where he ranked first in his class. Shortly after graduation he married Jean Munson and they had four boys who have degrees in electrical engineering or computer science.

From his early years he enjoyed projects using his hands and knew he wanted to be a surgeon. Interest in the nervous system probably came from the influence of his father, a professor in the child psychology department at the University of Iowa. This interest was solidified by an externship in neurology at the end of his freshman year when he came under the influence of Adolph

Sahs, Robert Utterback, and the chief resident at that time, Robert Joynt. This also provided his first introduction to research.

Realizing that he wanted to go into neurosurgery, he decided to take a rotating internship at the Cincinnati General Hospital to obtain a broad background in all aspects of medicine. Needing a year of general surgery he entered Dr. Michael DeBakey's program in Houston where he had an interesting and rewarding year of training.

On July 1, 1957 he entered the neurosurgical residency at the Massachusetts General Hospital (MGH) where he came under the influence of neurosurgeons James C. White, William Sweet, and H. Thomas Ballantine and the neurologists C. Miller Fisher, Raymond D. Adams, and Maurice Victor. After completing residency in 1961, he remained on the staff advancing to the rank of professor of surgery at Harvard Medical School and visiting neurosurgeon at the MGH. He was elected to a term as chairman of the staff associates, served 3 years on the General Executive Committee of the hospital, and has been a member of several hospital Committees.

Over the years at the MGH he has enjoyed teaching a group of outstanding residents and working with a superb staff. His publications include over 150 articles and two books that centered in the earlier years on his interest in cerebrovascular disease. More recently his clinical activities have been directed toward benign tumors particularly acoustic neuromas and meningiomas. He has been asked to give numerous invited lectures and has been a visiting professor at many institutions.

His first job with the Congress came when John Shillito approached him to be an assistant editor for *Clinical Neurosurgery*. Subsequently, he became the editor of that publication. Later Bill Mosberg asked him to be nominated for the Executive Committee and he remained on that committee for 11 years including a 3-year term as secretary.

During his presidential year in 1975 to 1976 the first joint officers meeting between the Congress and the American Association of Neurological Surgeons (AANS) was held, plans were finalized for publication of *Neurosurgery*, and the Washington Committee became a reality. The years on the Congress Executive Committee were both challenging and rewarding. Friendships were made that continue to this day. As he looks back on that era he believes that the opportunity for the young neurosurgeon to be active in national affairs is an important strength for neurosurgery in this country.

In 1977 he began a 6-year term on the American Board of Neurological Surgery serving as chairman in 1982 to 1983. His term on the Board of Directors of the AANS started in 1982 and he was president of the Association in 1986 to 1987. A highlight of the term was a ceremony at the White House where President Ronald Reagan announced the printing of a stamp to honor Harvey Cushing. Subsequently, he was president of the American Academy of Neurological Surgeons and of the Society of Neurological Surgeons.

Membership in other medical organizations include the Massachusetts Medical Society, American Medical Association, American College of Surgeons, and the New England Neurosurgical Society. He was a founding member and served as president of the Society of University Neurosurgeons.

Nonmedical interests include spending time with the family, stamp collecting, hiking, landscaping, carpentry work, and tennis. In addition he has served as a deacon in his church and both he and his wife feel a strong commitment to their beliefs. He has often stated that he feels most fortunate to have had a rewarding and interesting life.

1977

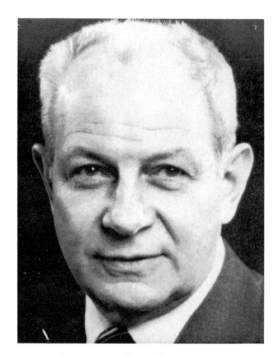

RICHARD COY SCHNEIDER

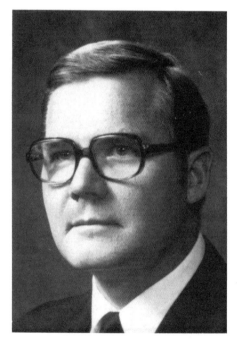

BRUCE FARRELL SORENSEN

Richard Coy Schneider

Richard Coy Schneider was born in 1913 to Dr. and Mrs. Louis Schneider in Newark, New Jersey, where his father, having trained at the University of Pennsylvania, was a general practitioner. He attended Culver Military Academy, graduated in 1931, and then became an undergraduate at Dartmouth, where he was active in both lacrosse and swimming. One of his hobbies was traveling, and he satisfied this, as well as the need for some extra money, by working summers on freighters on the Old Dollar-Line. The first summer he traveled to the Mediterranean, and during the next he was head pantry man on a ship that traveled around the world, despite a strike on the part of most of the crew, with Dick leading the strikebreakers. Thus, as a teenager in those times, he had seen a good bit of the world. After receiving an A.B. degree from Dartmouth, he sought and gained entrance to the University of Pennsylvania Medical School, receiving his M.D. in 1939. Between his junior and senior years, he worked on a dude ranch where he and the other ranch hands would anesthetize horses with chloral hydrate and "do the shoeing."

He returned home for an internship at Newark City Hospital and took a year in pathology at Cleveland City Hospital and a year of surgery at Detroit Receiving Hospital, where he was a fellow studying contaminated wounds under a National Research Council project. In 1943, he married Madeline T. Thomas of Finley, Ohio. They had courted for a number of years, despite their geographic separation, with Madeline attending Bryn Mawr and working at the Massachusetts Institute of Technology and Dick at Dartmouth and then the University of Pennsylvania. Shortly thereafter, he had to report to the Carisle Barracks, and during World War II he served in North Africa, Italy, and France on the neurosurgical service of the 36th General Hospital under Lieutenant Colonel John Webster. During this period he became chief of neurosurgery at the 236th Hospital and consultant at the Percy Jones Hospital. Following the war, he went to the University of Michigan at Ann Arbor for his neurosurgical training under Dr. Max Peet, practiced neurosurgery for several years in Cleveland, and then at the invitation of Dr. Edgar Kahn, in 1950, he returned to Ann Arbor as an assistant professor. He became an associate professor in 1952 and professor in 1962. He began the neurosurgical service at St. Joseph's Mercy Hospital. When Doctor Kahn retired in 1969, he became chief of the Section of Neurosurgery at the University of Michigan.

Dr. Schneider's bibliography includes extensive publications on head and cord injuries. He described the mechanisms of acute central cord injury and hangman's fracture and made important observations concerning the role of vascular insufficiency of the brain stem due to injury to the neck and spinal column. In addition to his book documenting serious and fatal football injuries, he was coeditor with Drs. Kahn and Crosby of the first and second editions of *Correlative Neurosurgery* and served as editor of an expanded third edition. Later in his career, he edited a definitive reference on sports injuries. His association and research efforts with Dr. Elizabeth Crosby spanned a quarter of a century and included studies on the interplay between the cerebral hemispheres and cerebellum in relation to abnormal movements, as well as tonus. Together, they studied rotational movement patterns associated with vestibular centers in the brain stem and have contributed to the understanding of the role of association bundles in producing clinical and electroencephalographic signs at a distance from the actual lesion site.

Dr. Schneider was a tireless worker capable of long hours in the hospital, office, and laboratories. His ability to be involved in and to finish many simultaneous projects was recognized not only in Ann Arbor, but nationally. Thus, as well as his membership and activities in the Congress of Neurosurgeons (CNS), he was a member of the American College of Surgeons, American Medical Association, Association for Research in Nervous and Mental Diseases, American EEG Society, American Association of Neurological Surgeons (AANS), Neurosurgical Society of America, American Academy of Neurosurgery, Neurosurgical Travel Club, and American Association for Surgery of Trauma. He had many committee assignments and held many national posts. Among them, he was president of the AANS in 1974 and was on the Board of Directors between 1970 and 1977, and he was a member of the American Board of Neurosurgery between 1966 and 1972 and was vice chairman between 1970 and 1972. In addition, he served as a visiting professor in institutions in this country and abroad.

Doctor Schneider was first and foremost, a teacher and was able to transmit enthusiasm for neurosurgery not only to house officers but also to students. He was also able to delegate both patient care and operative responsibility; yet he supervised in such a way that the house officer learned not only by watching but also by doing. Although his extensive neurosurgical activities did not permit him much free time, he enjoyed swimming at the Barton Hills Country Club and long walks. He shared with his wife a love for travel, having visited 60 countries in his lifetime. His wife, Madeline, was a strong factor in his success and is an avid gardener and homemaker and also finds time to serve as a volunteer at the University Hospital. Dr. Richard Schneider died June 9, 1986.

DAVID G. KLINE, M.D.

Bruce Farrell Sorensen

Bruce Farrell Sorensen was born January 25, 1931 in Aurora, Illinois, the second son of Alton H. Sorensen, Sr. and Ruth Bergquist. His father had just completed a master's degree in structural engineering at the University of Illinois when Bruce was born. Shortly thereafter, the family moved to Salt Lake City, Utah where two more sons and a daughter joined the family.

Bruce attended Salt Lake City schools where he distinguished himself in athletics as an All-State football player and was president of his high school àcapella choir. He attended the University of Utah on an athletic scholarship but his football career was cut short with injuries and subsequent surgery on both knees. Bruce was declared ineligible for military service during the Korean War because of his knees and was therefore able to fulfill a mission for the Church of Jesus Christ of Latter-Day Saints.

After his mission he resumed his education at the University of Utah. He served as the president of the chapter of Sigma Chi fraternity and graduated with a B.S. degree in 1956. Two days after graduation, Bruce and Suzanne Kirkham Burbidge were married. That fall, they moved to Philadelphia where Bruce attended Temple University School of Medicine. During those years, two sons were born to the Sorensens, John Burbidge and Stephen Bruce. Bruce graduated from Temple University School of Medicine in 1960. Bruce was president of both his junior and senior classes and was invited to join the Babcock Surgical Society. During his senior year, he came under the influence of Dr. Michael Scott, professor of neurosurgery at Temple, who stimulated his interest in neurological surgery.

Bruce returned to Salt Lake City and served 1 year in a general rotating internship followed by 1 year of residency in general surgery. A third son, Scott Kirkham was born. Bruce then became a fellow in neurosurgery at the Cleveland Clinic in Cleveland, Ohio training with Drs. W. James Gardner, Wallace B. Hamby, and Donald F. Dohn. Bruce returned to Salt Lake City after he completed his residency in neurological surgery and has remained in the private practice of neurological surgery since that time. A fourth son, Evan Burke, and finally a daughter, Elizabeth, were added to his family. Shortly after Bruce completed his residency, Dr. Donald Dohn, one of his mentors insisted he join the Congress of Neurological Surgeons (CNS). During his first year in the CNS he served on the Host Committee. He then became committee chairman and next chairman of the Registration Committee. After 3 years on the Executive Committee he was elected treasurer of the CNS. Bruce was president in 1976. His year as president culminated in the Congress meeting in San Francisco with Dr. Richard C. Schneider serving as the honored guest. One of the highlights of his year as president was the publication of the first volume of *Neurosurgery* under the editorship of Dr. Robert H. Wilkins. That year there was expansion of the Socio-Economics Committee with inclusion of representatives of all state neurosurgical societies at the annual meeting and closer ties with the American Association of Neurological Surgeons (AANS) were fostered. At the conclusion of his year as president of the Congress, he was elected to the Board of Directors of the American Association of Neurological Surgeons and after 3 years became the treasurer of the AANS. He has served on several committees of the AANS. He recently was chairman of the Ethics Committee during which time the Association's ethics codes were written and adopted. His most recent assignment has been as chairman of the Professional Conduct Committee of the AANS. Dr. Sorensen is a Fellow of the American College of Surgeons and served on the Advisory Counsel for Neurosurgery. He is also a member of the Society of Neurological Surgeons, Western Neurological Society, and the Rocky Mountain Neurosurgical Society.

Finding time for church service has always been a part of the Sorensen family life. Bruce has served in many leadership capacities including bishop counselor, bishop, and as a member of a three-man Stake Presidency, overseeing the activities of 10 congregations of church members exceeding 4,500 members. Family activities include travel, hunting, fishing, and hiking in the mountains. Bruce has a keen appreciation for wilderness areas and loves nothing more than an opportunity to enjoy nature. At the present time Bruce and Suzanne have nine grandchildren.

1978

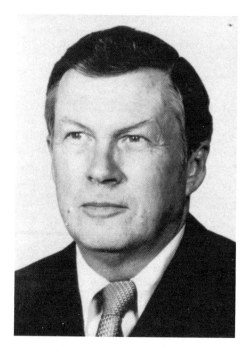

CHARLES GEORGE DRAKE

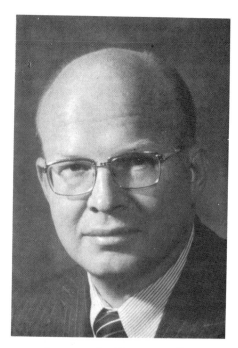

ALBERT L. RHOTON, JR.

Charles George Drake

Charles George Drake was born on July 21, 1920, and received his early education in Windsor, Ontario. A teacher remembers Charlie as "the most thoughtful and determined student" he had ever known, and these personality traits perhaps more than anything else characterize the man and his career. At the age of 18, he moved to London, Ontario, and graduated in 1944 from the Faculty of Medicine at the University of Western Ontario. He initially planned a career in internal medicine but while interning at the Toronto General Hospital a senior resident became ill, and Charlie was recruited to be the only houseman on the neurosurgical service. This contact with the Toronto School of Surgery and that quiet genius of Canadian neurosurgery, Kenneth G. McKenzie, changed the direction of his life. Drake was fascinated with McKenzie the surgeon, and drawn to McKenzie the man, for they had much in common, a passion for fishing and the outdoors, a natural athletic ability, and a contemplative determination in their approach to a problem. McKenzie, a general surgeon converted late to neurosurgery, recognized the need for fundamental training in neurobiology and influenced Drake to begin his training in the growing field of neurophysiology, culminating in a year with John Fulton at Yale University. During this year Drake studied the functional motor localization of the cerebellum. A year of general surgery with Angus McLaughlin was followed by 2 years of clinical training with McKenzie and Botterell on the busy Toronto General neurosurgical service, where he learned the art and craft of neurosurgery. McKenzie and Botterell recognized the exciting future in the surgical treatment of intracranial aneurysms and arteriovenous malformations (AVM) and encouraged Drake to seek solutions to the then many unsolved problems in their management.

During this period, Charlie courted and married a beautiful student nurse, Ruth Pitts. In 1951, he, Ruth, and their first child, John, traveled to Great Britain to study neurology at the National Hospital at Queen's Square and to meet and observe the leading neurosurgeons of Europe of the time, including Sir Hugh Cairns, Norman Dott, Gustav Norlen, and Herbert Olivecrona.

In 1952 Drake returned to London against the advice and conventional wisdom of many, as the first and for some years the only neurosurgeon in Southwestern Ontario. He joined the staff of the Faculty of Medicine at the University of Western Ontario, where his natural ability, sound training, and the continued support of Professor Angus McLaughlin (who he was to succeed as the chairman of the Department of Surgery 22 years later) ensured success. He was soon recognized as an excellent neurologist and a bold and uncommonly skillful surgeon. His practice flourished, but he avoided the hazard of being overwhelmed and diverted by the large number of cases by training general surgeons and orthopedists to assist in the care of patients with trauma of the nervous system. Working alone, he was early to recognize the need for expert associates. In Paul New, and later John Allcock, he was fortunate to have the guidance and assistance of two of the pioneers of modern neuroradiology. In Ronald Aitken, he had a gifted and perceptive anesthetist who developed and perfected many of the techniques which permitted the direct attack on many heretofore unapproachable vascular lesions of the nervous system. Appreciating the enormous resources he had in the many patients under his care, Drake worked diligently at new approaches and new solutions to old problems, meticulously perfecting his technique and carefully recording his results. Out of this effort came a series of publications, in 1978 numbering more than 70, covering a wide breadth of neurosurgery, characterized by lucid technical descriptions and a candid, honest style which emphasized failures as well as triumphs.

It was the intracranial aneurysm and AVM that were to become the focus of his energies, and for the next 25 years he set a standard for the world in the treatment of these common and deadly lesions. Drake, Allcock, and Aitken furthered our understanding of aneurysms and subarachnoid hemorrhage with their astute observations on vasospasm, the tragedies of early operation, the important of magnified vision and postoperative angiography, and the safety and limits of intentional, deep hypotension to make the exposure and dissection safe and even possible. In 1978, he had operated on more than 1000 aneurysms and since his first attack on a superior cerebellar artery aneurysm in 1958 to 1978, he had operated on more than 600 aneurysms arising from the vertebral-basilar system. By 1978, he had operated on more than 150 AVMs, and his success in dealing with aneurysms and AVMs of all sizes and at all sites is unparalleled. It is perhaps more important that he has openly shared the triumphs and tragedies of his large surgical experience and thereby assisted the development of this exciting field for all neurosurgeons.

These surgical accomplishments would suffice for most men, but Charlie was early recognized by his peers as a leader and spokesman. He has given unselfishly of his time and effort to neurosurgery, surgery, and the community of medicine. He has been president of the Royal College of Physicians of Canada, president of the American Association of Neurological Surgeons, president of the World Federation of Neurological Surgeons, president of the Canadian Neurosurgical Society, member of the Board of Regents of the American College of Surgeons, chairman of the Editorial Board of the *Journal of Neurosurgery*, and visiting professor and guest lecturer in most of the countries of the world. These duties have been carried out with good humor and wisdom while maintaining a demanding and rigorous neurosurgical practice.

Perhaps his most proud professional achievement, however, was the development of the Department of Clinical Neurological Sciences at Western. In 1969, Drake and his longtime friend Henry Barnett joined Neurosurgery, Neurology, Neuropathology, and Neuroradiology into one cohesive unit. This department, now the second largest in the medical school, has effectively removed the artificial barriers between medical and surgical neurology to provide the optimum care for patients and a foundation for clinical and basic research into neurologic disease.

What makes Drake unique? Of course, he possesses those qualities necessary in every surgeon. He has good hands and excellent surgical technique, not dainty or flashy but solid and workmanlike. He has an uncanny perception of surgical anatomy and is able to decipher the most complex anatomical situation, even in the most confining exposure, with apparent ease. He is a good neurologist. He is capable of exceptionally hard work and possesses unusual stamina which enables him to operate on 8 or 10 major cases every week and stand at the operating table for 10 or 12 hours and still be able to work at the same pace at the end of the case as he did at the beginning. He has always set a high standard for himself and for others to keep good records. He has kept handwritten notes and drawings on every major case that he has operated upon, highlighting the clinical history and physical findings and the details of the operation, postoperative course, and follow-up. These running track sheets, assembled into large looseleaf books, have been the foundation for the published reports of results over the years.

Perhaps his most unique characteristics which distinguish a great neurosurgeon from the rest are his single-mindedness and determination. He is able to concentrate and return again and again to a problem until a solution is found. He is not easily dissuaded by the attempts and failures of others or what at first appears to be an impossible situation. Moreover, he is able to learn and grow from an error, adversity, and apparent defeat. When one looks back over his pioneering efforts in the surgical treatment of aneurysms and AVMs of the posterior circulation, one realizes that most of us would soon have given up, for there were many early disasters. But success surely depends on reflection, perseverance, endurance, and the ability to start up fresh and enthusiastic after each disappointment. Charlie brings a large measure of all of these qualities to every problem.

For those of us who have had the privilege of working with Charlie, he is known as a wise physician, intuitive neurologist, and a superb, decisive neurosurgeon. He is determined to push back the frontiers of neurosurgery by thoughtfully responding to new and different ideas. He continually asks "How can we do this better?" while stressing safety, reason, and judgment.

Charles Drake is a man of many interests and diverse skills. He handles his airplane, shotgun, fly rod, and squash racquet with the same care, dexterity, and enthusiasm with which he handles an aneurysm clip. He has enjoyed marvelous support from his gracious and understanding wife and lively family. He and Ruth have raised four fine sons and proudly exclaim the virtues of their two grandsons.

It was a privilege to recognize Charles Drake as the honored guest of the Congress of Neurological Surgeons, for he in turn adds distinction and honor to this organization.

SYDNEY J. PEERLESS, M.D., F.R.C.S.(C)

Albert L. Rhoton, Jr.

Albert L. Rhoton, Jr. was born November 18, 1932, in Parvin, Kentucky. He graduated from Washington University School of Medicine, *cum laude*, with the highest academic standing in the class of 1959. As a medical student, he did research on the trigeminal nerve and on cerebellar electrophysiology.

He had 2 years of training at Columbia-Presbyterian Medical Center in New York, one year in general surgery and 1 year in neurological surgery. He returned to Washington University and Barnes Hospital where he completed his neurosurgery residency with Dr. Henry Schwartz in 1965. He stayed at

Washington University for 1 year as a research fellow in neuroanatomy. At this time he began to use the microscope for his research work and immediately saw that it would be very useful for work in human neurosurgery.

In January 1966, Dr. Rhoton went to the Mayo Clinic where he served as a consultant and staff neurosurgeon, and began his microanatomical studies of human material that are now so widely published. In 1972, he assumed the position of professor of surgery and chief of the Division of Neurological Surgery at the University of Florida College of Medicine. The Division was awarded departmental status and he became the R.D. Keene Family Professor and Chairman of the Department of Neurological Surgery in 1981. His departmental associates, under his guidance, have grown to be recognized as authorities in the subspecialties. He has obtained funds for eight $1 million endowed chairs in neurosurgery at the University of Florida.

Dr. Rhoton became a member of the Executive Committee of the Congress of Neurological Surgeons (CNS) in 1972 and rose to presidency of the Congress in 1978. He served as annual meeting chairman in 1973. A major goal during his presidency was to strengthen the relationship of the national and state neurosurgical societies. In pursuit of this goal, the first of a series of annual meetings between officers of the state and national neurosurgical societies was held in 1978 in Washington, D.C. at the Congress Meeting over which he presided. He also played a key role in the founding of the Joint Section on the Spine of the American Association of Neurological Surgeons (AANS) and CNS. During the time that he was president of the Congress, there was a tremendous surge of interest in cerebrovascular surgery and at that time he served as chairman of the Joint Section on Cerebrovascular Surgery. Dr. Charles Drake of London, Ontario served as the honored guest at the 1978 meeting in Washington, D.C. At that time, Dr. Rhoton experienced a gnawing discomfort because cerebrovascular and intracranial surgery overshadowed spinal neurosurgery. As president of the Congress, he expressed these concerns and proposed the development of a spine section which was later approved by both the AANS and CNS and eventually became one of the strongest Joint Sections.

Dr. Rhoton has earned numerous honors and awards throughout his career. He served as president of the American Association of Neurological Surgeons in 1990 and as vice chairman of the American Board of Neurological Surgery in 1991. Washington University School of Medicine recognized his many accomplishments by awarding him an Alumni Achievement Award in 1984. He has been the honored guest or honorary member of 16 neurosurgical societies throughout the United States, Latin America, Europe, Asia, and Africa.

He organized a microsurgery course in Gainesville, Florida that has been attended by more than 1000 practicing physicians and residents. The University of Florida recognized his service by giving him the Distinguished Faculty Award in 1981. He has served on the editorial boards of six journals.

Dr. Rhoton has been supported and greatly aided by his wife, Joyce. Their two sons are resident physicians, one in internal medicine and the other in neurosurgery. Their two daughters are also in medicine, one as a pediatric nurse and the other as a resident in obstetrics and gynecology.

1979

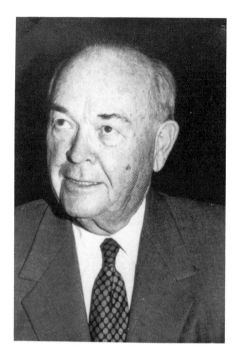

Frank Henderson Mayfield

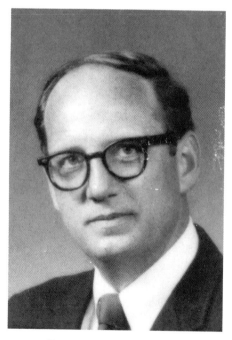

David L. Kelly, Jr.

Frank Henderson Mayfield

Frank Henderson Mayfield was born on June 23, 1908, and spent his early years on a farm in Garnett, South Carolina. Formative experiences imbued him with a sense of duty and historical perspective evident to all who have encountered his imaginative and logical mind.

When Frank was 12, the Mayfield family moved back to the ancestral home in North Carolina where his interest in farming and his considerable skills as an athlete were developed. He might have remained near the soil had his wise and gentle mother not stimulated him to enroll in the University of North Carolina and then the Medical College of Virginia. Her untimely death, a month before his graduation in 1931, was a grievous occasion for the young physician.

Frank planned a career in public health, but fortunately his talents attracted the attention of Dr. Claude Coleman, a pioneer in neurosurgery at the Medical College of Virginia who played a major role in his development and subsequent eminence in neurosurgery. Dr. Coleman was highly regarded by both Drs. Cushing and Dandy, a tribute to his courtly manner, fidelity, and surgical skill, characteristics that were revered by his protégé, Frank Mayfield. During his association with Dr. Coleman and in visits to the clinics of Drs. Cushing and Dandy, Frank was able to assimilate much of the laudable teachings of both schools of this rapidly evolving profession.

During his training Frank was attracted to the genteel loveliness and character of the operating room supervisor, and in 1936 the same Queenee Jones became his wife. In the years since their marriage Queenee's charming countenance graced and complemented her dynamic husband: her forbearance, faith, and finesse enabled her to raise their four children in much the same way their paternal grandmother had raised hers.

In 1935, Dr. Coleman arranged for Frank to join Dr. Glen Spurling as an associate and teaching assistant at the University of Louisville. An immediate friendship developed between them and Dr. Mayfield's interest in the spine, kindled by previous association with Dr. Crutchfield in Virginia, was stimulated. Observations concerning the lumbar disc, the ligamentum flavum, and the effective space in the spinal canal were potent indicators of evolving contributions. At this time there was little understanding of the nature of degenerative disorders of the spine, and the mortality associated with cranial surgery was prohibitive in many hospitals of the South and Midwest. When most medical schools were seeking the services of qualified neurological surgeons, Frank Mayfield, aged 29, moved to Cincinnati, Ohio, to establish a community practice of neurological surgery. In Cincinnati, a synergistic relationship was struck between Frank Mayfield and Joseph Evans, director of the Department of Neurosurgery at the University of Cincinnati College of Medicine, and between the community hospitals and the University of Cincinnati. This mutual respect and cooperation led to the development of a residency training program which nurtured the investigative concepts of Dr. Penfield and the clinical-surgical principles of Drs. Cushing and Dandy, and elevated Frank Mayfield to the rank of clinical professor of surgery (neurosurgery) at the University of Cincinnati.

Departments of Neurosurgery that were to prosper for 40 years under Dr. Mayfield's direction were established at the Christ and Good Samaritan Hospitals. This partnership was interrupted only once, when from 1942 to 1945, Dr. Mayfield was called to serve as chief of neurosurgery at Percy Jones General Hospital, Battle Creek, Michigan. Here his interest in spinal and peripheral nerve injuries were published.

On returning to Cincinnati, Frank's ability as a clinician, his organizational talents, and his gifts of certitude and friendship led to meteoric recognition as a surgeon, administrator, and educator. The basis for corporative practice was established, a concept later emulated throughout the country; collaboration with George Kees, a talented medical artist, led to the development of the paradigm for arterial aneurysm clips and other surgical instruments. As chairman of the Subcommittee on Crash Injury Prevention, and the first neurosurgeon to serve the Committee on Trauma, American College of Surgeons, he collaborated with Mr. Fletcher Platt of the Ford Motor Company in the development of seat belts for automobiles. At home, he was sequentially elected president of the Ohio State Neurosurgical Society in 1947, the first chartered state neurosurgical society; the Academy of Medicine of Cincinnati, and the Ohio State Medical Association; and he was appointed to the Board of Directors of the University of Cincinnati. In 1958, Frank was appointed to the American Board of Neurological Surgery, became its chairman in 1962, and was voted a Distinguished Service Award in 1969. When, in 1964, Frank and his colleagues wisely perceived that American neurosurgery did not possess a unified voice, he as president of the Harvey Cushing Society proclaimed that henceforth the American Association of Neurological Surgeons would be that spokesman. Despite Frank's humble disavowal of personal credit for the many honors bestowed upon him, his ethics, vision, prodigious energy, and his total regard for the sanctity of friendship led his peers to call him "the neurosurgeon's neurosurgeon" and the "conscience of neurosurgery."

He was honored by his colleagues in Ohio with an honorary Doctor of Science Degree from the University of Cincinnati in 1971 and as the Neurosurgeon of the Year in 1967. In 1977 he was selected as the first recipient of the Harvey Cushing Medal by the American Association of Neurological Surgeons. The American Medical Association bestowed upon him The Distinguished Service Award in 1980.

Frank had the uncanny ability to know everything that was going on about him. His close alliance with members of the political and business world and his innumerable affiliations with the legal, religious, educational, and journalism fields enabled him to serve a wide variety of causes and councils with distinction and exactness. Frank's firm commitment to the "tribal rule" accredits the sanctity of physician-patient relationships; his determination to make himself and his colleagues worthy of the respect and confidence of the public and his opposition to the encroachment of outside authorities on the prerogatives of the profession earned him unique respect from his fellow men. The Congress of Neurological Surgeons was privileged to recognize Frank H.

Mayfield as its honored guest, for he was the friend of all neurosurgeons. Dr. Frank Mayfield died January 2, 1991.

JOHN M. TEW, JR., M.D.

David L. Kelly, Jr.

David L. Kelly, Jr., was born in Elkin, North Carolina, April 25, 1935. He received his undergraduate degree from the University of North Carolina. He was elected to Phi Eta Sigma and Phi Beta Kappa. He graduated from the University of North Carolina Medical School having been elected to Alpha Omega Alpha in 1959. He received his neurosurgical training at Bowman Gray School of Medicine/North Carolina Baptist Hospital in Winston-Salem, Children's Hospital and Peter Bent Brigham Hospital in Boston, and did a fellowship in neurophysiology at Washington University in St. Louis. In 1965 he joined the faculty at Bowman Gray and was promoted to professor in 1978. In 1979 he was made chairman and head of the Department of Neurological Surgery at Bowman Gray.

Dr. Kelly's major clinical and neurosurgical interests are in vascular malformations of the brain, spine stabilization, pituitary and acoustic tumors, and tic douloureux. His major academic interests are in resident education and training, as he has served as chairman of a committee for the Society of Neurological Surgeons to do a longitudinal study of resident selection and evaluation.

Dr. Kelly served for 6 years on the American Board of Neurological Surgery. After having participated in organized neurosurgery for a number of years, he served on the Board of Directors of the American Association of Neurological Surgeons (AANS), then as secretary, vice president, and president from 1990 to 1991. He served as secretary and then president of the Congress of Neurological Surgeons, and has also chaired many of its committees. He served as vice president of both the Neurosurgical Society of America and the Southern Neurosurgical Society.

Dr. Kelly has over 100 publications to his credit, and he has served on a number of editorial boards. He received the Distinguished Service Award from the University of North Carolina in 1990. At the present time, he remains chairman and head of the Department of Neurological Surgery and occupies the Eben Alexander Chair of Neurological Surgery.

During his years of leadership with the Congress of Neurological Surgeons, a Certification Committee of the Congress was established which was designed to assist those individuals who had not been successful in passing the oral examination by the American Board of Neurological Surgeons. That program was extremely successful in terms of having a high percentage of candidates receive their certificate following intensive study and preparation. Also, during his year as president of the Congress, the American Association of Neurological Surgeons extended an invitation to the Congress to become amalgamated with the AANS. The Executive Committee felt that move would not be in the best overall interest of neurosurgery. The AANS and the Congress jointly formed a Spine Section which rapidly became one of the most active and important sections in neurological surgery. The Joint Socio-Economic Committee gained stature and recognition within the Congress of Neurological Surgeons to the point that they became an integral part of the decision-making and issue discussion process. There was some discussion as to whether the Joint Socio-Economic Committee should perhaps become aligned with the Congress, but it was felt that the major role of the Congress should be in education and development of the young neurosurgeon.

1980

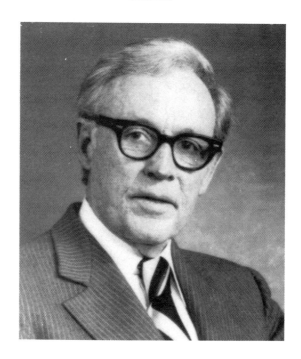

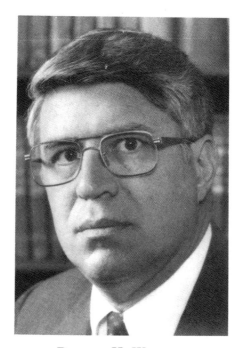

Robert H. Wilkins

Eben Alexander, Jr.

Dr. Eben Alexander, Jr., was born on September 14, 1913, to Dr. and Mrs. Eben Alexander, Sr., of Knoxville, Tennessee, where Dr. Alexander was a prominent general surgeon. Eben, Jr., attended the University of North Carolina and received his A.B. degree at Chapel Hill, where his grandfather was a professor of Greek. He then went on to Harvard Medical School, receiving his M.D. degree *cum laude* in 1939. Among his classmates were Drs. John Adams, Kenneth Livingston, Francis Moore, and the late and beloved Dr. Donald Matson. Dr. Alexander is the permanent president of the class of 1939 and served as the president of the Harvard Medical Alumni Association for 1980 and 1981.

Dr. Alexander was attracted into neurological surgery by Dr. Franc Ingraham, who was his teacher and great friend. Dr. Ingraham, one of the finest and most respected gentlemen in neurological surgery, had a great influence upon Dr. Alexander's career.

Dr. Alexander's internship and residency at Peter Bent Brigham and Children's Hospital in Boston spanned a 9-year period from 1939 to 1948, being interrupted by World War II. He returned from the war with a rank of major, the Bronze Star, and a great appreciation for the comforts of home. His home fires had been lit when he married Elizabeth West in 1942. Betty has been a source of strength for him. Her graciousness and charm are appreciated by members of many neurosurgical organizations, by civic groups, and by their many friends.

Dr. Alexander was fortunate enough to serve a year of neurosurgical residency from 1948 to 1949 under Dr. Kenneth McKenzie in Toronto, Canada. That year was rewarding to Dr. Alexander, not only because he was exposed to Dr. McKenzie's outstanding skills but also because he had the opportunity to review Dr. McKenzie's series of patients with 8th nerve tumors. That published review represented the state of the art at that time.

In 1949, Dr. Alexander was appointed assistant professor of surgery in charge of neurological surgery and in 1954 became professor and head of the Section on Neurological Surgery, Bowman Gray School of Medicine of Wake Forest University. He held this position until October 1978. As director of the neurosurgical program, he was responsible for the training of 31 residents. His emphasis on the clinical practice of neurosurgery caused his program to be recognized as one of the best in the nation.

From 1953 through 1973, Dr. Alexander served as chief of Professional Services of North Carolina Baptist Hospital. During that period the medical center in Winston-Salem grew, and much of the present prominence of both the Bowman Gray School of Medicine and North Carolina Baptist Hospital is the result of his efforts and leadership.

Dr. Alexander's contribution to neurological surgery, both at the laboratory and clinical levels, is documented in over 100 publications. His research projects have focused on hydrocephalus, peripheral nerve injuries, craniosynostosis, spinal cord injuries, and brain tumor chemotherapy. He was one of the first neurosurgeons to recognize the value of plastics in neurosurgery. His clinical interests cover a wide range of subjects, but most often have related to cranial and spinal injuries, brain tumors, and intracranial aneurysms. He has maintained his interest and enthusiasm for pediatric neurosurgery by continuing to contribute to the surgical treatment of many congenital lesions.

His influence on organized neurosurgery at the national level has been truly remarkable. He has made contributions to the National Institutes of Health and the American Association of Medical Colleges. He has served as president of the Society of Neurological Surgeons, the American Academy of Neurological Surgeons, and the American Association of Neurological Surgeons. He served on the Executive Committee of the American Association of Neurological Surgeons and was an officer from 1959 to 1967 when he became president of that association. He also served on the editorial board of the *Journal of Neurosurgery* from 1961 to 1970.

For the past few years, Dr. Alexander has made a great effort on our behalf in the American Medical Association (AMA). He has participated in the development of the AMA Section Council for Neurosurgery. He has also served on the Interspecialty Advisory board, the Council of Medical Specialty Societies, and the Council on Medical Education. He has recently been appointed to the National Board of Medical Examiners and the Liaison Committee for Graduate Medical Education.

Dr. Alexander has earned the respect of all neurosurgeons. For those who have had the privilege of knowing him well for many years, he is appreciated for his attention to detail, demand for excellence, compassion and dedication to his patients, positive and optimistic attitudes, honesty and fairness in all endeavors, and for his perseverance and commitment to organization and progress.

He earned the privilege to be recognized as the honored guest of the Congress for 1980.

DAVID L. KELLY, JR., M.D.

Robert H. Wilkins

Robert H. Wilkins was born in Pittsburgh, Pennsylvania, on August 18, 1934. He received the B.S. degree from the University of Pittsburgh in 1955 and the M.D. degree from the same institution in 1959. He received his postgraduate training at the Duke University Medical Center (2 years of general surgery and 5 years of neurosurgery), spending the 2 years between these segments as a clinical associate in the Surgery Branch of the National Cancer Institute in Bethesda, Maryland. Following the completion of his residency, Dr. Wilkins joined the neurosurgical faculty of Duke University and was an assistant professor from 1968 through 1972. The next 4 years were spent as chairman of the Department of Neurosurgery at the Scott and White Clinic in Temple, Texas (3 years) and as associate professor in the Department of Neurological Surgery at the University of Pittsburgh (1 year). Dr. Wilkins then returned to Duke University where he has been professor and chief of the Division of Neurosurgery since 1976.

Dr. Wilkins has published more than 230 medical papers and chapters and has edited and authored a total of nine books. From 1975 to 1976 he was an associate editor of *Surgical Neurology*. He is currently on the editorial boards of the *Journal of Neurosurgery*, *British Journal of Neurosurgery*, and *Acta Neurochirurgica*. Dr. Wilkins has been active in several neurosurgical organizations, including the American Association of Neurological Surgeons of which he is treasurer, and the Southern Neurosurgical Society of which he is a president-elect. He is currently a member of the National Advisory Council on Neurological Disorders and Stroke.

Dr. Wilkins joined the Congress of Neurological Surgeons in 1969 and took part in various committee activities. He was a member of the Congress Executive Committee from 1973 to 1976 and was president from 1979 to 1980. As part of his duties for the Congress of Neurological Surgeons, Dr. Wilkins was editor of *Clinical Neurosurgery* from 1972 to 1975 and was the founding editor of *Neurosurgery* from 1977 to 1982.

During his year as president of the Congress of Neurological Surgeons, the business of the organization went on as usual. However, the site of the 1980 Annual Meeting had to be switched at the last minute from Miami because of the deterioration of the conditions at the hotel with which the initial contract had been set years before. The Congress was fortunate to find excellent accommodations in Houston and the meeting went off without incident. The scientific program included a segment on the preparation and presentation of scientific material. Dr. Frank Netter gave a memorable talk on medical illustration in which he did not show a single slide or make use of any other visual material; furthermore, his speech, which was recorded and transcribed, required virtually no editing to prepare it for publication in *Clinical Neurosurgery*!

1981

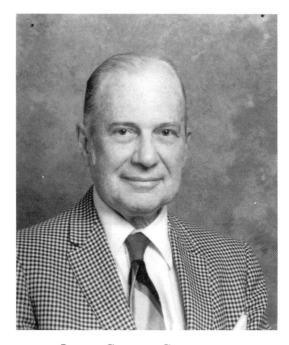

JAMES GARBER GALBRAITH

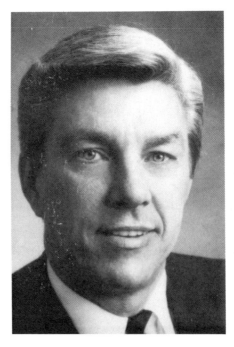

JAMES FLETCHER LEE

James Garber Galbraith

James Garber Galbraith was born in 1914 in Anniston, Alabama. He was the first son of Mr. and Mrs. Samuel Love Galbraith. His father, a banker, was a quiet, retiring man and, before his marriage, a Presbyterian. His mother Sadie was a petite, vivacious, well-loved Southern lady, a devout Catholic who set a first-class table. Her father, Dr. James Rhodes Garber, Sr., was one of the early physicians in Alabama. Garber, his brother Wilfred, and his sister Mary were all reared in their mother's religion. Garber was an excellent student at St. Bernard's and fell in love with golf at a young age. He was influenced early in his life towards a medical career by his mother's twin brother, Dr. James Rhodes Garber, Jr., a prominent obstetrician in Birmingham. Indeed, as his uncle's namesake, Garber was almost obliged to pursue a medical career.

After high school, he attended the University of Notre Dame from 1930 to 1932 and subsequently received his B.S. degree and M.D. degree from St. Louis University, graduating from the School of Medicine in 1938. He interned at the Lloyd Noland Hospital in Fairfield, Alabama and remained for a year of general surgery. One of his friends recalled that Dr. Galbraith routinely had a big party for his friends and fellow physicians every Labor Day and asked his guests to bring their own food and drink. After the party, he allegedly had enough spirit to last until his next Dutch-treat party.

He went for his neurosurgical training to the New York Neurological Institute at Columbia Presbyterian Medical Center, completing his training there in 1943. He entered the Navy in 1943 and was assigned to New Orleans. Subsequently, he was transferred to Guadalcanal and, upon completion of his naval duty, returned to medical practice in neurological surgery in Birmingham, where he enjoyed an active private practice and served as the neurosurgeon at the University. He assisted in the training of Dr. Stanley Graham, his first partner, and subsequently formed an association with Dr. Griff Harsh and others in an outstanding neurosurgical group. He remained in charge of the neurosurgical training and the private practice from 1946 to 1965. He became associate professor of Neurological Surgery at the University of Alabama School of Medicine in 1946 and became professor and director of the Division of Neurosurgery in 1954. As professor of Neurosurgery at the Medical School, he was pleased at the appointment of his long-time colleague and associate, Dr. Griff Harsh, as director of the training program in 1978.

His academic honors include membership in Alpha Omega Alpha and Alpha Sigma Nu. He received the Alumni Merit Award from St. Louis University in 1973 and the Citation for Distinguished Service from Columbia University in 1967. In addition, in 1974, he received the honorary degree of Doctor of Humane Letters from St. Bernard College. Dr. Galbraith has had many medical honors, locally, regionally, and nationally. He was president of the Jefferson County Medical Society in 1960 and president of the Medical Association of the State of Alabama from 1974 to 1975. He has been president of the Southern Medical Association, Southern Neurosurgical Society, American Academy of Neurological Surgery, Society of Neurological Surgeons, and chairman of the American Board of Neurological Surgery. He served as a member of the Board of Governors of the American College of Surgeons from 1974 to 1980 and has long been a member of the American Association of Neurological Surgeons. In addition, he is so well respected by his peers that he served as a member of the Board of Censors for the Medical Association of the State of Alabama from 1969 to 1976. He has been active in public service in Birmingham, both as a member of the Board of Directors of the Chamber of Commerce and as a member of other public service boards.

In addition to training a host of neurosurgeons, his scientific contributions consist of publications concerned with cerebral aneurysms, cerebral occlusive disease, brain tumors, and craniocerebral trauma. His area of expertise is craniotomy for meningioma. One of his residents has stated that Dr. Galbraith occasionally has shown the influence of profanity-inducing hemostasis, particularly with a difficult meningioma. Throughout his career, he has demonstrated a devotion and contribution to neurological surgery in every aspect imagined. As a clinical neurosurgeon, he is known as a man of great common sense and decisive action.

He is married to Marguerite Stabler Galbraith, affectionately known as Peggy. They have been blessed with four daughters, Ann, Jane, Kay, and Laura, and in 1981 had three granddaughters and a grandson. Dr. Galbraith has maintained his interest in golf and has long been a member of the Mountainbrook Country Club in Birmingham. Every Wednesday afternoon has been reserved for golf for as long as his associates can remember. He is so intent on his game that allegedly he played golf with an old friend on two or three occasions during which time the friend was developing a mild hemiparesis with a subdural hematoma. Garber's pride at his repeated victories over this friend during this period were suddenly deflated.

His medical achievements represent the contributions of an outstanding clinical neurosurgeon. Of equal importance are his personal attributes. He is the epitome of the Southern gentleman. He has a wonderful combination of humility and common sense tempered by intelligence. He has the unique ability to disagree without appearing to disagree. He has been a counselor to neurosurgeons young and old in the South. He has the ability to listen, immediately determine the problem, and quickly and compassionately offer good advice and solutions. There are numerous stories of his counseling; perhaps one of the best is exemplified by the story of a frustrated new program director from Tennessee who asked to speak to Dr. Galbraith about adopting or developing a sense of direction. He was immediately invited to stop by Birmingham, picked up at the airport, enjoyed a sandwich in the quietness of Dr. Galbraith's office, returned to the airport with a firm handshake, and departed with renewed purpose and a workable solution to his problems.

Throughout all of his activities, Dr. Galbraith has been an ardent gardener, particularly with roses but also with vegetables. He secretly has been a fan of W. C. Fields for many years. He appreciates ladies and has a unique way of letting them know it. He enjoys dancing and most social events. The Congress was proud to have Dr. J. Garber Galbraith, gentleman, physician, surgeon, counselor, leader, teacher, and friend, as its Honored Guest in 1981.

James Fletcher Lee

James Fletcher Lee, the second of three sons, was born in the historical southern city of Murfreesboro, Tennessee in 1934, where his parents, Jack and Mary Lee, raised him, along with his two brothers, in the Methodist religion. He and Mrs. Lee instilled in their children the importance of honesty and integrity and encouraged the desire to excel in whatever projects came one's way. Fletcher always enjoyed his schoolwork and in high school additionally enjoyed sports, primarily basketball and football, though the former was his choice. A football injury dampened this interest, but at the same time, opened another avenue, which for some time held such a strong attraction, that it seemed destined to be his life profession.

No longer involved in sports, Fletcher obtained a job at the local airport, where his pay was awarded in flying time. At age 16, he soloed and obtained his student pilot's certificate, and at 17, his private pilot's certificate. At 18, he obtained his commercial pilot's certificate and flight instructor's rating, and seemed well on the road to his chosen profession. He elected to attend the University of Tennessee in Knoxville, and was fortunate to be awarded there an instructor position with the University of Tennessee Flight Training Program. He found that this was too time-consuming and detracted from his college studies. After completing his first year in college, he obtained summer employment at the hospital in Murfreesboro, Tennessee. This seems to have been the point in his life when his interest turned to medicine.

The beautiful campus of the University of Tennessee at Knoxville became the incubator for his second and still-compelling interest in life, medicine. Graduating from the University of Tennessee *cum laude*, with an A.B. degree in zoology, and having served as president of Alpha Epsilon Delta, the honor premedical society at the University, Dr. Lee next attended Duke University School of Medicine. He regards those 4 years as some of the happiest in his life. He graduated from medical school in 1960 and, in that year, was elected to Alpha Omega Alpha, and was the recipient of the C.V. Mosby Scholarship Award.

With his interest still primarily in general surgery, Dr. Lee entered a surgical internship at Duke. During that year and the year of general surgery assistant residency that followed, he came under the influence of Drs. Barnes Woodhall and Guy Odom and the neurosurgical program at Duke. While in the second of those 2 years, he visited other neurosurgical programs but elected to remain at Duke for his neurosurgical training, under these two outstanding physicians. He next spent a year on medical neurology, then proceeded to neurosurgery, completing that season of his professional growth as chief resident in neurosurgery, in 1966 to 1967. During most of that time, he served in the United States Army Reserve retiring as major.

Upon completion of his neurosurgical residency, Dr. Lee moved to San Antonio and established a private practice of neurological surgery and in 1969 obtained certification by the American Board of Neurological Surgery. He has greatly enjoyed private practice, particularly relishing the direct patient contact and the opportunities for interaction with and care of his patients thus provided. He has had the good fortune to be in close proximity to the University of Texas Health Science Center at San Antonio, and holds the title there of clinical professor of neurological surgery.

It was during his early years in private practice that Dr. Lee saw the opportunity to become active in the Congress of Neurological Surgeons and in so doing, to meet and interact personally with other neurosurgeons throughout the country, allowing him the chance to consult with them regarding patient management problems. Beginning initially with committee tasks, he first became treasurer and then president. In his year as president of the Congress of Neurological Surgeons, his primary goal was to oversee the development of an outstanding annual meeting which was to be held in Los Angeles, California. He was very ably assisted in this by Drs. Fletcher Eyster, annual meeting chairman; Chris Shields, scientific program chairman; and Martin Weiss, local arrangements chairman. Also, as in previous years, the Congress and the American Association of Neurological Surgeons were attempting to unite some of their activities and goals, in order to provide a more unified and effective management of them. Significant time was devoted to investigating and promoting these amalgamations.

In addition to these honors, Dr. Lee held the position of alternate delegate to the American Medical Association from the Congress and served on the Board of the Alamo Heights United Methodist Church. Having held many staff positions at Southwest Texas Methodist Hospital, he assumed the post of chief of staff in 1984. Dr. Lee presently is on the Board of the Bexar County Medical Society, the Advisory Board of Hospice San Antonio, and the Board of Ecumenical Center for Religion and Health, where he is second vice president.

During his training and in subsequent years, Dr. Lee has contributed articles to the medical literature and served as editor of a book entitled, *Pain Management.*

Throughout his life, he has been blessed with a loving family and friends. This could never be more epitomized than by his lovely wife, Jane Volz Lee and their four beautiful daughters. In addition, there are now three lively grandchildren. In his spare time, he enjoys time with his family, as well as other activities including classical music, fly fishing, and duck decoy carving.

1982

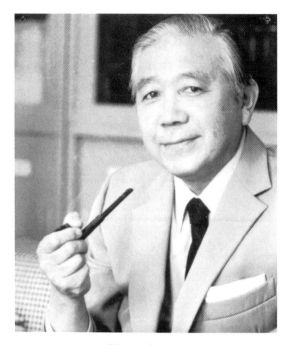

Keiji Sano

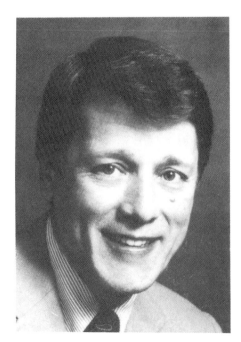

Donald H. Stewart, Jr.

Keiji Sano

Dr. Keiji Sano was born on June 30, 1920, in the quiet and scenic town of Fujinomiya in Shizuoka Prefecture which lies at the foot of Mt. Fuji, about 100 kilometers to the west of Tokyo. He was the first son of Dr. and Mrs. Takeo Sano. His father was a well-known surgeon. After Dr. Sano graduated from high school there, he entered the University of Tokyo Faculty of Medicine, from which he graduated with his M.D. degree in 1945.

Because there was no internship in Japan, he joined the First Surgical Department of the University of Tokyo to receive postgraduate training in general surgery from Professor Ohtsuki. Neurosurgery in Japan originated from this department of surgery through the efforts of Kentaro Shimizu (1903–). Dr. Shimizu first joined the Department of Psychiatry after graduating from the University of Tokyo in 1929, but when two of his patients died from misdiagnosed brain tumors, he changed his mind and became a neurosurgeon. In 1932, he joined the First Surgical Department. When Dr. Sano joined the Department, Dr. Shimizu was actively practicing neurosurgery as an associate professor of surgery.

In 1948, Dr. Shimizu became the professor and chairman of the First Surgical Department and, thereafter, Dr. Sano specialized in neurosurgery. In 1948 he published several papers on the techniques of percutaneous cerebral angiography. In 1951, he was awarded a degree of Doctor of Medical Science (D.M.Sc.); which corresponds to a Ph.D. in medicine. Dr. Sano obtained a fellowship from the Ministry of Education of Japan to study neurosurgery with Drs. Naffziger and Boldrey at the University of California at San Francisco and neuropathology with Dr. Nathan Malmud from 1951 to 1952.

Dr. Sano was promoted to lecturer and chief of the outpatient clinic of neurosurgery in 1955 and then to associate professor of neurosurgery at the Institute of Brain Research, University of Tokyo Faculty of Medicine, in 1957. In the same year he was married to his wife, Sumako. In 1962 the Japanese Government first approved and opened an independent department of neurosurgery at the University of Tokyo and appointed Dr. Sano as the first professor and chairman of the department. Later in the same year, another department of neurosurgery was approved at Niigata University where Dr. Komei Ueki was appointed as the professor and chairman. Drs. Sano and Ueki, pioneering neurosurgeons, worked continuously for almost half a century until neurosurgery was officially recognized as a definite independent discipline of clinical medicine. An additional 10 years were necessary until the Japanese government decided to open a department of neurosurgery in every national university hospital.

In 1948, the first meeting on neurosurgical research was held at Niigata, and after seven meetings, the Japan Neurosurgical Society was organized in 1952. In 1965, Dr. Sano was elected the president of the Japan Neurosurgical Society. In addition to being the secretary for the society for 20 years of his professorship, he devoted his entire professional life not only to his own neurosurgical research at the University of Tokyo but also to the development of neurosurgery throughout Japan by establishing a standardized postgraduate training curriculum for neurosurgery.

The Japanese Board of Neurosurgery was organized in 1966 with regulations on training curriculum and training institutes; Dr. Sano was the chairman of the board from 1967 to 1973 and again from 1979 to 1980. He was also the president of the Japanese Association for Research in Stereo-Encephalotomy in 1966, president of the Asian and Australasian Society of Neurological Surgeons from 1967 to 1971, president of the World Federation of Neurosurgical Societies from 1969 to 1973, chairman of the 3rd Conference on surgery of Apoplexy in 1974, president of the Japanese Society of CNS Computed Tomography since 1978, general chairman of the Workshop on Pituitary Tumors since 1978, chairman of the 3rd Wilder Penfield Memorial Conference in 1980, president of the 4th Conference on Neurotraumatology in 1981, and president of the Japanese Congress of Neurological Surgeons in 1981.

His contribution to neurosurgical research has been outstanding. Between 1948 and 1981, he published 629 papers (153 in English and 2 in German), including 162 on intracranial and spinal tumors, 119 on cerebrovascular diseases, 80 on head injuries, 48 on stereotactic and functional neurosurgery, 43 on EEG, 32 on other diagnostic methods, 24 on congenital anomalies and pediatric neurosurgery, 20 on operative techniques and paraoperative care, and 16 on epilepsy.

Obviously, the scope of his research has been too wide to review here. I would like to make special mention, though, of his works on thalamotomy for pain, posteromedial hypothalamotomy for pain and behavior disorders, BUdR-antimetabolite-radiation therapy and boron-neutron capture therapy for glioblastoma, and artificial embolization for large AVMs, and his research on the mechanism of vasopasm and of head injuries.

It is with the great pride of all Japanese neurosurgeons that Dr. Keiji Sano, the real establisher of Japanese neurosurgery, was invited to be the honored guest of the 32nd Annual Meeting of the Congress of Neurological Surgeons.

KENICHI UEMURA

Donald H. Stewart, Jr.

Donald H. Stewart, Jr. was born a "Tar Heel" at Duke University Hospital on December 8, 1934. His family lived in Chapel Hill, North Carolina, but there was no hospital there at the time. His father, a Presbyterian minister, had immigrated to this country from England in the 1920s. They lived for awhile in Frankfort, Kentucky where he attended the first grade. In April 1941 they moved to Houston, Texas where Dr. Stewart graduated from high school and then he returned to North Carolina to attend Davidson College. He subsequently attended Washington University School of Medicine.

After 2 years of medical school, he thought that perhaps research would be more interesting and applied for and received a National Institute of Health fellowship that enabled him to spend a year in London at St. Thomas' Hospital before returning to complete his medical degree in St. Louis. A year of medical internship at Duke with Dr. Eugene Stead and then a year of general surgery with Dr. Nathan Womach at the University of North Carolina was highlighted by Dr. Stewart marrying Anne Donnelly who was a senior at Duke University. Dr. and Mrs. Stewart moved to Syracuse so he could study neurosurgery under the tutelage of Drs. Robert King, Herbert Lourie, and Sidney Watkins. After spending 2 years in the United States Air Force (1968–1970), they returned to Syracuse where Dr. Stewart entered the practice of neurosurgery and he and Anne raised their four children.

Dr. and Mrs. Stewart were pleased when he was asked to be president of the Congress as he had not moved up through any elective office but, rather, had spent considerable time working with the Joint Socio-Economic Committee as well as the Washington Committee of which he was a founding member. They resumed the custom of having the June Executive Committee Meeting at a location where it would be suitable for their families to join them in the off hours so they could combine work with vacation. This resulted in a much more pleasant and fraternal group and led to the development of many long-term friendships.

Since the annual meeting was to be held in Toronto, they made a special effort to become acquainted with Canadian neurosurgeons and involve them in the Congress. They were particularly pleased that Susan and Alan Hudson spearheaded this planning effort and they since have become great friends. They count many other Canadians as close friends as well.

Dr. Stewart tried to create an international flavor for the Congress and invited Dr. Keiji Sano, an eminent Japanese neurosurgeon, to be the honored guest. This greatly facilitated further friendships and dialogue between North American and Japanese neurosurgeons.

Since those days in the early 1980s, their children have grown, married, finished college, and medical school and they, too, have continued to enjoy life and the many associations made as a result of their time with the Congress of Neurological Surgeons. Dr. Stewart has spent several years on the Board of the American Association of Neurological Surgeons (AANS) along with other former Congress presidents, and currently serves as the vice president of that organization. To his great enjoyment, Dr. Stewart was reappointed to the Washington Committee. He has also served as chairman of the Guidelines Committee of the AANS which developed the first set of surgical procedure guidelines established on a national consensus basis. Currently he is the chairman of the Peer Review Committee of the AANS which is attempting to establish a peer review system for neurosurgery.

1983

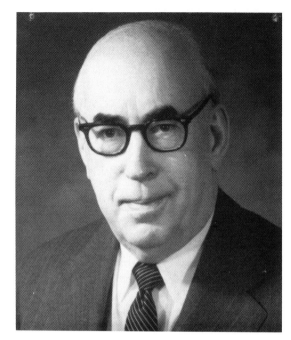

C. MILLER FISHER

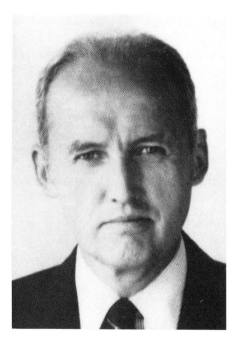

JOHN M. TEW, JR.

C. Miller Fisher

The remarkable accomplishments of C. Miller Fisher, astute observer and describer of clinical phenomena, pathologist, investigator, dedicated physician, and teacher have been summarized in two publications commemorating C. Miller Fisher Day, which was held on September 7, 1980, at the Massachusetts General Hospital (1, 2). It is appropriate on this occasion to review the life of this outstanding physician.

C. Miller Fisher (CMF) was born in the small town of Waterloo, Ontario, Canada, on December 5, 1913. By the time he reached age 10 it was assumed by his family that he would become a doctor, and no thought was ever given to any other career. Following graduation from high school he entered Victoria College in the University of Toronto, where he enrolled in a special 7-year course which combined a science B.A. and M.D. program. While accomplishing an outstanding academic record, he was a member of the University swimming and water polo teams.

Following graduation from medical school in 1938, he won a highly competitive internship at the Henry Ford Hospital and then in 1939 went to the Royal Victoria Hospital in Montreal as a medical resident. World War II was looming, and in April of 1940 he entered the Navy but in a somewhat unusual fashion. A naval surgeon on the staff of the Royal Victoria Hospital applied for transfer but could only do it if he could find another physician to replace him in the Navy. CMF volunteered and divided his time between the residency and examining recruits. After France fell, the call came for volunteer surgeon-lieutenants to go to England, and Dr. Fisher went on loan to the royal Navy in September 1940. His assignment was as a general medical officer at the Portsmouth Naval Base on the south coast of England, with his time being divided among medical care, training for defense against a possible invasion of England, and running to air raid shelters.

After a few months he was placed as a medical officer on a cruiser patrolling the North Atlantic Ocean near northern Scotland, Iceland, and Greenland. After spending several dark winter months in this area, his ship docked at Halifax, Canada, for a planned rest period. Hardly had he come ashore when the doctor on another cruiser that was about to leave became ill. CMF took his place, leaving Halifax almost immediately and headed for the South Atlantic. Early in the morning of April 4, 1941, while steaming toward Africa, his cruiser was engaged in surface action by a German raider and sunk. Nine hours were spent in the water before he was picked up by the German vessel. He was transferred to a prison ship and was eventually taken to a prison camp in northern Germany, where he stayed for 3½ years.

In this camp he served as a medical officer for prisoners. Two events during this period probably influenced his career. He learned to read German, which enabled him in later years to study the very important original German literature on cerebrovascular disease. He also was able to read widely on many subjects—history, English literature, mathematics, navigation, etc. which not only occupied his time but, he believes in retrospect, satisfied the yen that all of us have to enjoy a great intellectual feast as adults rather than as fledgling students. Thus, he was able to devote his time to medicine without feeling that all else had passed him by.

In September 1944, he was sent back to Canada during the repatriation of prisoners and was assigned to the naval hospital in Halifax. At about this time it was realized that CMF had not had the benefit of a period of specialized training which the Canadian government had been giving medical officers serving in the Forces. Under this program he returned to the Royal Victoria Hospital to continue his training in medicine, with a special interest in endocrinology and diabetes. During this time he had a 2-month rotation on neurology at the Montreal Neurological Institute (MNI), and it was here that one clinical case and one man, Dr. Wilder Penfield, changed the direction of his career. A United States Army general entered the MNI with a seizure disorder, which included the history of hearing the beat of tom-toms, followed by loss of consciousness. CMF recounts that he knew nothing about this clinical problem, so he decided to get out the books. Elementary sleuthing suggested a tumor localized in Heschl's gyrus. Apparently Dr. Penfield was impressed and asked if CMF had considered neurology as a career. A position as acting-registrar of the MNI was offered and accepted. During the next 2 years at MNI he developed an interest in hypertensive encephalopathy and conducted a careful follow-up study on 103 patients who had had a lumbodorsal sympathectomy for hypertension. At the end of this 2-year period, Dr. Penfield proposed that he go abroad for further training in cerebrovascular disease. Dr. Roy Swank felt strongly that there was only one person with whom to train, Dr. Raymond D. Adams at Boston City Hospital. CMF went to Boston on January 1, 1949, spending the next year in neuropathology and enjoying the teaching of both Dr. Adams and Dr. Denny-Brown.

This was his first experience with morbid anatomy, and his interest became centered in cerebrovascular pathology. One of his first observations was that while most of the clinical diagnoses of stroke patients from the general medical services were "middle cerebral artery thrombosis," this was rarely the finding when the brain was examined. Often he had to examine five or six brains per day, sometimes more. One afternoon he was to cut 10 brains. The first had a hemorrhagic infarction, but dissection of the vessels revealed no occlusion. Brain five had another hemorrhagic infarction and, again, no vessel occlusion was found. Late in the afternoon, a third brain had the same findings. At that time relatively little was known about the dynamics of cerebral embolism, and such findings were said to be due to vasospasm. When he looked at the clinical records on all three of these patients, it was found they were atrial fibrillators. When he inspected the distal arterial branches, small emboli particles were found. In this one afternoon the whole idea of the migration, lysis, and disappearance of emboli was formulated, and the relationship of embolism to hemorrhagic infarction was demonstrated. It is of interest that when this finding was first written up, it was not accepted for publication by any pathology journal. It was this study that started him reading the German literature, which emphasized to him how little was known about the vascular pathology in cerebrovascular disease.

CMF returned to the Montreal General Hospital in 1950, where he was to spend the next 4½ years. Three individuals were important to him during this time. He was under the tutelage of Dr. Francis MacNaughton, who was the prime mover in starting a clinical stroke program. At that time, hospital admission of stroke patients was discouraged, but Dr. MacNaughton overcame this problem. Dr. Harold Elliott, the neurosurgeon, was extremely cooperative and encouraged the venture in every way. Last but not least, Dr. Lyman Duff, dean and professor of pathology at McGill, gave strong support to the development of cerebrovascular neuropathology.

Shortly after returning to Canada, CMF had occasion to examine a patient with a stroke at the Veterans Hospital. This is when the concept of transient ischemic attacks (TIA) got started. The patient said, "It is remarkable, before I became paralyzed I would go blind in one eye off and on for just a short time, but when I got paralyzed it was on the wrong side." Within 2 weeks another patient came with the same story. CMF, on looking up the literature, found that a persistent blindness in one eye and permanent paralysis on the opposite side meant carotid occlusion. The idea that hemiplegia and transient monocular blindness might be due to carotid stenosis was born. Several months later the first TIA patient died from metastatic carcinoma when CMF was out of town. When he returned to find that no autopsy had been done, he learned that the family was willing, and with their permission, arrangements were made for it to be done in the funeral home at 11 p.m. the night before the funeral. For the first time, the clinicopathologic correlation of carotid occlusion and TIA was established. During the next 2 years he interviewed many stroke patients at a chronic hospital and one after another told of prodromal symptoms; he examined 1100 pairs of carotid and vertebral arteries for clinicopathologic correlations; and he developed the idea of using anticoagulant therapy to prevent stroke in patients with TIA.

Dr. Raymond Adams, who had by now been appointed chief of neurology at the Massachusetts General Hospital (MGH) and Bullard Professor of Neuropathology at Harvard Medical School, invited CMF to return to Boston to develop a stroke service and continue his cerebrovascular pathological studies. During his 3 decades at the MGH, CMF has continued to describe clinical phenomena, make clinicopathologic observations, teach, publish, and be a compassionate physician. Dr. Fisher's list of accomplishments is long. More than 90 of his publications relate directly to cerebrovascular disease, and many of the others relate to observations and ideas gained from examining stroke patients. Already mentioned are the clinicopathologic correlations in cerebral embolism and carotid artery atherosclerosis and the definition of TIA. Original observations have been made on the examination of the comatose patient, the distribution of atherosclerotic lesions in cervical and intracranial arteries, anatomic variations in the circle of Willis, the fundus oculi during an amblyopic attack, clinical and pathological study of lateral medullary infarction, pathology and clinical syndromes of brain hemorrhage, early diagnosis of all types of stroke patients, the clinical syndrome of small thalamic hemorrhage, the diagnosis of cerebellar hemorrhage, anatomical vascular lesions causing the lacunar state, lacunar syndromes, inflammatory vascular disease, facial pulses in carotid occlusion, carotid bruits, vasospasm in association with ruptured saccular aneurysm, dissection of the internal carotid artery, late life migraine, capsular infarcts, ocular bobbing, transient global amnesia, normal pressure hydrocephalus, and a number of other clinical and pathological problems. His description of Creutzfeldt-Jakob disease made possible the diagnosis in life.

He originated many descriptive terms, some of which are part of our everyday vocabulary. These include TIA, transient monocular blindness (TMB), subclavian steal, symptomatic normal pressure hydrocephalus, the "string" sign, transient global amnesia, lipohyalinosis, transient migraine accompaniments (TMA), pure motor hemiplegia, pure sensory stroke, ataxic hemiparesis, dysarthria-clumsy hand syndrome, ocular bobbing, and the one-and-a-half syndrome.

What are the factors that allowed almost 3 decades of an exceptionally productive career? First one must emphasize his long association at MGH with Dr. Adams, who gave him free rein in pursuing whatever activity CMF thought was fruitful. There are the 25 years of generous uninterrupted support from the National Institutes of Health, without which many of the contributions would not have been possible. An important factor for Dr. Fisher is his congenial working relationship with the neurosurgeons at MGH. His stroke fellows, however, were really the main instruments by which everything or anything was accomplished, as they took him in tow to see hundreds, indeed thousands, of stroke patients, always prodding with questions at CMF and not infrequently raising a skeptical brow. Day in, day out, there was the excitement of finding something new or puzzling on every patient. CMFs first fellow was Herbert Karp and then followed: Carl Bridges, Irving Zeiper, Ernest Picard, John Barlow, Alfred Weiss, Mercy Sodka, Alfred Polak, Jean Angelo, Monro Cole, Jean-Pierre Berger, Proful Dalal, Hiram Curry, Jay Mohr, Louis Caplan, Otto Appenzeller, and Laurent Des Carries. Rounds with his fellows would often last until midnight. CMF felt that clinical evaluation must be unhurried, and only in the evening was there time to spend with patients in a leisurely fashion.

Of great importance to CMF's career has been the support of his lovely wife, Doris, to whom he has been married for 44 years. She has helped him in every way possible, has not complained about his long hours, and has allowed him to devote full efforts to the unsolved problems of neurology. She says it is a team effort.

Anyone fortunate enough to work with this dedicated physician will be aware of his unique approach to clinical neurology. Every discussion of a patient's problem is a learning experience, for each case will be reviewed in relationship to his vast background. His ability to organize clinical observations into well-ordered patterns has led to a method and style that has been a constant inspiration. Dr. Lou Caplan has summarized into "Fisher's Rules" the basic principles CMF has followed in his approach to medicine (2):

1. The bedside can be your laboratory. Study the patient seriously.
2. Settle an issue as it arises at the bedside.
3. Make a hypothesis and then try as hard as you can to disprove it or find the exception before accepting it as valid.
4. Always be working on one or more projects; it will make the daily routine more meaningful.
5. In arriving at a clinical diagnosis, think of the five most common findings (historical, physical, or laboratory) found in a given disorder.
6. Describe quantitatively and precisely.
7. The details of the case are important; their analysis distinguishes the expert from the journeyman.

8. Collect and categorize phenomena; their mechanism and meaning may become clearer later if enough cases are gathered.

9. Fully accept what you have heard or read only when you have verified it yourself.

10. Learn from your own past experience and that of others (literature and experienced colleagues).

11. Didactic talks benefit most the lecturer. We teach others best by listening, questioning, and demonstrating.

12. Write often and carefully. Let others gain from your work and ideas.

13. Pay particular attention to the specifics of the patient with a known diagnosis; it will be helpful later when similar phenomena occur in an unknown case.

14. Be a good listener; even from the mouths of beginners may come wisdom.

15. Resist the temptation to prematurely place a case or disorder into a diagnostic cubbyhole that fits poorly.

16. The patient is always doing the best he can.

17. Maintain a lively interest in patients and people.

Even though CMF has reached "retirement age," Dr. Joseph Martin, chief of neurology, has provided him an office to continue his clinical and pathological studies. He can still be found pondering a patient's clinical problem, reading in the library, or looking at slides late into the evening hours. As a member of the MGH neurosurgery service, I feel very fortunate to be working with this "neurosurgeon's neurologist."

ROBERT G. OJEMANN, M.D.

REFERENCE

1. Adams, R. D., and Richardson, E. P. Salute to C. Miller Fisher. Arch. Neurol., *38*: 137–139, 1981.
2. Caplan, L. R. Fisher's rules. Arch. Neurol., *39:* 389–390, 1982.

John M. Tew, Jr.

Dr. John M. Tew, Jr. began his education at Wake Forest University and the Bowman-Gray School of Medicine. Completing his early surgical training at Cornell Medical Center and Peter Bent Brigham Hospital, Dr. Tew spent 2 years as a clinical associate at the National Institutes of Health and the Armed Forces Institute of Pathology in Bethesda, Maryland. He completed his neurosurgical training at Massachusetts General Hospital and Boston Children's Hospital. In 1969, Dr. Tew was awarded the William P. Van Waggen Fellowship in Neurosurgery and studied at the University of Zürich with Professor Gazi Yasargil.

In 1973, Drs. Tew and Thor Sundt co-founded the Cerebrovascular Section of the American Association of Neurological Surgeons (AANS) and the Congress of Neurological Surgeons (CNS). Dr. Tew served as chairman in 1978. The section was established to promote and advance education, foster research, and improve patient care of diseases of the cerebrovascular system.

Committed to educational excellence, Dr. Tew was instrumental in developing the Physician's Recognition Award in Neurosurgery, established in 1975. Dr. Tew developed the mechanism for the AANS/CNS Joint Committee of Education to accredit courses, enabling physicians to receive category I credits for continuing education in neurosurgery.

In 1976, the AANS/CNS central office was initiated under the auspices of an Ad Hoc Committee, spearheaded by Dr. Tew, to meet growing demands for administrative coordination, bookkeeping, registration, neurosurgical communication, management of the annual meetings, and to serve as a central meeting facility. As chairman of the Joint Education Committee in 1979, Dr. Tew directed the committee's vision and development of the first self-assessment examination in neurological surgery, the SESAP-SANS.

Characterized by concern for medical competence, education, research and ethics, Dr. Tew served as president of the Congress of Neurological Surgeons in 1983. On behalf of neurosurgeons throughout the nation, Dr. Tew testified before the Senate Subcommittee on Labor, Health and Human Services, Education and Related Agencies Appropriations in support of federal funding for biomedical research on stroke.

From 1982 to 1985, Dr. Tew served on the National Advisory Council for the National Institutes of Health and the National Institute of Neurological and Communicative Disorders and Stroke. He is also past president of the Ohio State Neurosurgical Society.

Currently serving as professor and chairman of the Department of Neurosurgery at the University of Cincinnati Medical Center, Dr. Tew is also co-director of the Skull Base Team for University Hospital and is chief of neurosurgery at University Hospital and Children's Hospital Medical Center.

Associated with the Mayfield Neurological Institute, Dr. Tew is an internationally recognized pioneer and authority on the medical applications of lasers. An author, teacher, and frequent guest lecturer, Dr. Tew travels extensively, addressing surgical treatment of vascular tumors and arteriovenous malfunctions, laser technology, the neuroscience revolution, skull base surgery, trigeminal neuralgia, and cranial nerve tumors.

A leader in the Greater Cincinnati community, Dr. Tew serves on the Board of Directors of the Union Central Life Insurance Company; on the Board of Trustees of Xavier University; and as chairman of the Citizens Committee for Drake Hospital. He chairs the fund drive for the Science Center at Xavier University; and is a member of fund drive committees for the National Conference of Christians and Jews and the United Way.

Dr. Tew married Susan Smyth on July 9, 1966. They have three children: Margaret, 24, a graduate in business from the University of Texas, Austin; John Matson, 22, a graduate in business from Miami University, Oxford, OH; and Neal, 20, a premedical student at Harvard University.

1984

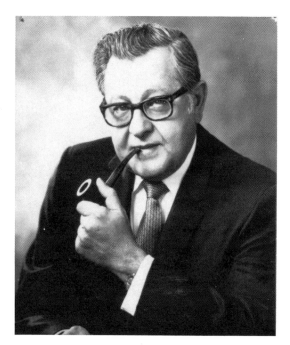

HUGO VICTOR RIZZOLI

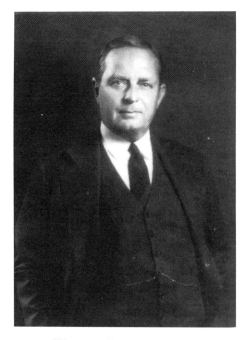

WALTER EDWARD DANDY

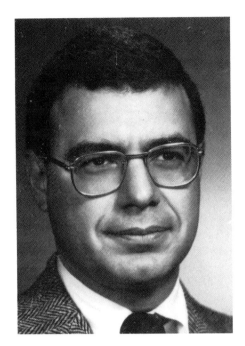

EDWARD R. LAWS, JR.

Hugo Victor Rizzoli

Hugo Victor Rizzoli was born in Newark, New Jersey, on August 20, 1916. He received his A.B. degree in chemistry from The Johns Hopkins University in Baltimore, Maryland, in 1936. Dr. Rizzoli then went on to receive his M.D. from The Johns Hopkins in 1940. He interned in medicine from 1940 to 1941, and then entered the surgery program at The Johns Hopkins. He became a Harvey Cushing Fellow from 1942 to 1943 and then served as neurosurgical resident with Walter E. Dandy as chief of service.

Dr. Rizzoli completed his residency during World War II and immediately entered the United States Army, serving as neurosurgeon at Halloran General Hospital and later at Walter Reed Army Hospital. Major Rizzoli served as chief of the neurosurgical section at Walter Reed for the year prior to his discharge from the Army in October 1946.

After leaving the Army, Dr. Rizzoli stayed in Washington, D.C., to practice neurosurgery. In addition to his private practice, he became chief of the Department of Neurosurgery at Emergency Hospital. Always a respected teacher, Dr. Rizzoli then became formally involved with the residency training program at the George Washington University. He had been chairman of the Department of Neurological Surgery and a member of the Board of Directors of the Washington Hospital Center, and was director of training and education there from 1964 to 1973. He was professor and chairman of the Department of Neurological Surgery at the George Washington University from 1969 to 1987.

Dr. Rizzoli's career has exemplified neurosurgery in the nation's service. He has been deeply involved with the Veterans Administration and has made numerous site visits to their spinal cord injury centers. He has continued to serve as consultant in neurological surgery to Walter Reed Army Medical Center, Bethesda Naval Hospital, Malcolm Grow Air Force Hospital, the Washington Veterans Administration Hospital, Andrews Air Force Base Hospital, and the National Institutes of Health. He was a member of the health exchange team of the Department of Health, Education and Welfare on a trip to the Soviet Union to study medical services for the treatment of spinal cord-injured patients. In 1979 he received the Department of the Army Commander's Award for Civilian Service which was presented by Walter Reed Army Hospital.

Many societies have had the benefit of Hugo Rizzoli's active participation. In the American Association of Neurological Surgeons he has served as vice president (1982), member of the Board of Directors and its Executive Committee, and chairman of the Graduate Education Subcommittee on Recertification of the Joint Committee on Education. He has been a member of the American Board of Neurological Surgery, has served as its vice chairman, and has served as Residency Review Committee member representing the American Medical Association. He represents the Society of Neurological Surgeons in the Association of Specialty Societies and Service Delegates and on the American Registry of Pathology. He is a member of the American Academy of Neurological Surgeons, the Neurosurgical Society of America (vice president in 1976–77), the American College of Surgeons, the Osler Society, the Clinical Pathological Society, and the Society of Medical Consultants to the Armed

Forces. He has been a member of the Congress of Neurological Surgeons since 1955.

Contributions to the medical literature have included his book on postoperative complications in neurosurgical practice, co-authored with Norman Horwitz and in its second edition, numerous articles on investigative work in spinal cord injury, earlier important papers on lumbar and cervical disc disease, peripheral nerve surgery, and the surgical management of aneurysms. His most recent contributions on the management of radiation necrosis of the brain continue to be both scientifically provocative and clinically useful.

Dr. Rizzoli and his wife, Helen Vargo Rizzoli, have four children, and they live in Chevy Chase, Maryland. Few neurosurgical educators have been as respected and beloved as Hugo Rizzoli. To the superb background in investigative and clinical neurosurgery he received from Walter Dandy, he has added his own brand of quiet and thoughtful excellence in practice, research, and education, and the Congress of Neurological Surgeons is privileged to honor him.

Walter Edward Dandy

Walter E. Dandy was born on April 6, 1886 in Sedalia, Missouri. His father was an engineer on the Missouri-Kansas-Texas Railroad. Dr. Dandy was an only child and maintained a close emotional relationship with his parents throughout his life. He was valedictorian of his high school class and the title of his commencement address was "Education." Dr. Dandy attended the University of Missouri where he was introduced to golf at the "near cow pasture golf course." Dr. Dandy developed a love for golf and played until the end of his life. However, Dandy had little time for recreation at the University. He helped defray his college expenses by working during the summers. He worked as a barn painter one summer and was a conductor and a motorman on a trolley line other summers.

Dr. Dandy enrolled in the University School of Medicine in his junior year and made straight As. He served as a student assistant to Dr. Jackson in the anatomy laboratory during his junior and senior years. He was elected to Phi Beta Kappa and also to Sigma Xi, the National Scientific Honorary Society. He graduated second in his class of more than 100 students on June 5, 1907.

Dr. Dandy applied to The Johns Hopkins School of Medicine for admission with advanced standing and was accepted into the second-year class beginning in the fall of 1907. Drs. Thomas Grover Orr and Raphael Eustace Semmes, Jr. were his classmates. The annual tuition was $200.00. Professor Franklin P. Mall was so pleased with Dandy's ability that he recommended him for membership in the American Association of Anatomists which was quite an honor for a second-year medical student. Dr. Dandy sought and obtained Harvey Cushing's consent to do research in the Huntarian Laboratory during his senior year in medical school. Following his graduation from Hopkins Medical School in 1910, Dr. Dandy became a Cushing Huntarian appointee for the year 1910 to 1911. Dandy became interested in the pituitary body and in 1911 he published an article with Dr. Emil Goetsch on "Blood Supply of the Pituitary Body." The beautiful drawings in this paper were made by Dandy, himself, under the coaching of Mr. Max Broedel, a renowned medical illustrator. Dandy received the master of arts degree in 1911 for his postgraduate work. He then entered the residency program at The Johns Hopkins Hospital as one of Dr. Cushing's assistant residents along with Howard C. Naffziger. Dr. Cushing was invited to become the professor of surgery at Harvard and surgeon-in-chief at the Peter Bent Brigham Hospital. Dr. Dandy had expected to be invited to go with Dr. Cushing. However, shortly before Cushing was to leave for Boston he came to the Huntarian Laboratory and asked to see Dandy's results on experiments with hydrocephalus. Dr. Dandy showed his work to Cushing and Dr. Cushing put it in a box of materials to take to Boston with him. Dandy took his work out of Dr. Cushing's box and told Cushing that the material was his and it was going to stay with him. Cushing then remarked that the work probably did not amount to anything anyhow. Shortly thereafter Dandy was informed that he was not being invited to go to Boston with Dr. Cushing.

Dr. William Halstead found a place on his staff for Dandy as an assistant resident surgeon as he was quite impressed with the research work that young Dr. Dandy and Dr. Kenneth Blackfan, a resident in pediatrics, were doing on hydrocephalus. Dandy performed his first craniotomy in 1912 while still on Dr. Cushing's service and he acquired considerable training and skill in general surgery. He felt that the best preparation for one wishing to become a neurosurgeon was to get a thorough training in general surgery first. Dandy's training at Hopkins lasted 8 years after his graduation from medical school. He undoubtedly contributed more to neurosurgery during his training period alone than any other neurosurgical resident.

Drs. Dandy and Blackman published their classical article on the origin, circulation, and absorption of cerebrospinal fluid and the production of experimental hydrocephalus in December 1913. Halstead stated that "Dr. Dandy will never do anything equal to this again. Few men make more than one great contribution to medicine." However, Dandy proved Dr. Halstead wrong. While still a surgical resident in 1918, Dandy introduced pneumoventriculography which became the most accurate diagnostic test for brain tumors for the next 50 years. Dr. Cushing's famous monograph on acoustic tumors was published in 1917 and he reported a case mortality rate of 18.1% and an operative mortality rate of 13.9% in 33 patients in whom he had performed a subtotal intracapsular removal. In that same year, Dandy performed his first successful total excision of an acoustic tumor. He later reported that in his last 41 cases of total extirpation by a unilateral approach, he had reduced his mortality to 2.4%. This was before the use of the surgical microscope. Dandy was the first to successfully remove a benign lateral ventricular tumor, an ependymoma localized by ventriculography. In October 1921 Dr. Dandy localized and successfully removed a colloid cyst of the third ventricle.

Dandy first performed section of the sensory root of the trigeminal nerve at the pons in 1925. He stated in his 1945 revision of *Surgery of the Brain* that 10% of his patients had either a tumor or an aneurysm as the cause of their tic douloureux. He stated that when a tumor was not present the etiology was almost always an arterial loop compressing and at times grooving the sensory root. Dr. Dandy performed this operation in more than 500 patients with less than an 0.5% mortality and with excellent and permanent relief of pain. Dandy felt that the attacks of vertigo in Meniere's syndrome were similar to the paroxysmal attacks that came with tic douloureux. He reported total section of the 8th nerve for Meniere's syndrome in nine cases in 1928 with the first case operated on in 1924. During his lifetime he did a total of 692 operations for Meniere's disease with only two fatalities and both of these were due to infection.

In 1929 Dandy reported two cases of L3 disc extrusion with back pain, bilateral sciatic pain, and cauda equina syndrome. A cisternal lipiodol myelogram was performed in both cases which demonstrated a complete block just above the L3 disc. Dandy operated on both patients, removed the fragments of disc, and both patients experienced excellent relief of pain. However, he did not pursue this subject further until after the famous contribution of Mixter and Barr in 1934. After that he became very enthusiastic about performing surgery on patients with herniated lumbar discs and operated upon more than 2000 patients without preoperative myelography.

In March of 1937, Dr. Dandy was the first to cure an internal carotid-posterior communicating artery aneurysm by occluding the neck of the aneurysm with a silver clip. His classic monograph *Intracranial Arterial Aneurysms* first appeared in 1944. He documented 133 aneurysms verified by operation or autopsy.

Dandy recognized the advantage of team work and he developed a "brain team." The 8-year surgical residency at Hopkins included 2 years of neuro-surgery rotations until 1941. Dr. Hugo Rizzoli reported that the members of the "brain team" held Dr. Dandy in awe and respect.

Dr. Dandy met Sadie Estelle Martin, a young attractive dietitian at The Johns Hopkins Hospital and after a 1-year romance married her on October 1, 1924. Dandy was 38 years old at the time and his bride was 23. During the first year of their marriage they took an art history course together at Goucher College. Besides operatic and symphonic performances, the Dandys enjoyed attending football games or baseball games. Exactly one year from the day of their marriage a son, Walter, Jr. was born. Walter Jr. was a medical student at The Johns Hopkins when Dr. Dandy died on April 19, 1946. The other children were Mary Ellen Dandy, born on July 22, 1927, Kathleen Louise Dandy, born August 29, 1928, and Margaret Martin Dandy, born January 21, 1935. The editorial in the Baltimore *Evening Sun* at the time of his death, summarizes well Dr. Dandy's contribution to neurological surgery: "He had imaginative genius to conceive of new and startling operative techniques, courage to try them, and skill, superb skill to make them successful."

Edward R. Laws, Jr.

Edward R. Laws was born on April 29, 1938 in New York City, the son of a physician. He left New York in 1955 to attend Princeton University where he received an A.B. with honors in the Special Program in American Civilization. He attended The Johns Hopkins School of Medicine (M.D. 1963), doing all of his elective work in the Department of Neurosurgery with studies on the histochemistry and cytochemistry of brain tumors. He stayed on at Hopkins to intern in surgery with Alfred Blalock, and after internship spent 2 years in the United States Public Health Service, assigned to the National Communicable Disease Center in Atlanta, and there was responsible for a research program in pesticide toxicology.

In 1966 he returned to The Johns Hopkins for residency training in neurosurgery under Dr. A. Earl Walker and joined the staff of The Johns Hopkins Hospital and School of Medicine in 1971 with initial major responsibility for pediatric neurosurgery. In September of 1972 he left Baltimore to join the staff of the Mayo Clinic and became deeply involved in pituitary surgery and epilepsy surgery, maintaining a research interest in the experimental biology of malignant brain tumors.

He married Peggy in 1962 after they met at The Johns Hopkins where she was working as an instructor at the school of nursing. They have four daughters and have worked closely together throughout their respective careers.

Ed became president of the Congress of Neurological Surgeons in 1984 with the annual meeting in New York City. It was decided to make Walter Dandy a posthumous honored guest and to have Hugo Rizzoli be the honored guest, with Hugo having been one of Dr. Dandy's most prominent residents. The meeting was a great success and it was particularly enjoyable to have it in a city known so well to Ed and Peggy. The highlights included a cocktail party for 2300 people on the aircraft carrier, *Independence*, and a presidential reception at the newly renovated Museum of Modern Art. At that time the Congress was making a major move to become an international organization and there were many participants from other countries. During the cocktail party on the aircraft carrier, the West Point Glee Club entertained.

Ed became the recipient of an endowed chair at the Mayo Clinic and then became editor of *Neurosurgery*. He and Peggy have worked together on the journal and she serves as the managing editor using her maiden name, Margaret Anderson.

In 1987 Dr. Laws had the opportunity to succeed Hugo Rizzoli as professor and chairman of the Department of Neurosurgery at the George Washington University Medical Center in Washington, D.C. He has worked hard there to build a superb residency training program based on a scientific approach to a wide spectrum of problems in clinical neurosurgery.

1985

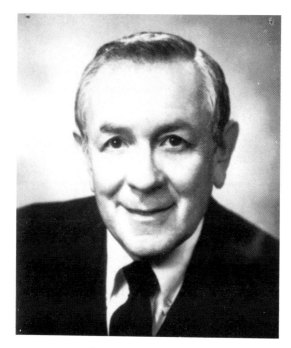

SIDNEY GOLDRING

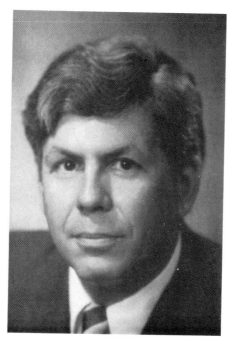

ROBERT A. RATCHESON

Sidney Goldring

Sidney Goldring was born April 2, 1923, in Kremnitz, Poland. His family immigrated to the United States and settled in St. Louis when Sidney was 3 months old. The Goldrings spoke not a word of English, but they had a passionate determination that their sons would be educated and have a profession. David, the first-born son, fulfilled his parents' dream by going to medical school. They, however, despaired of their second son, who was not distinguishing himself in school, and seemed more concerned about having fun and winning swimming meets for Soldan High School than getting serious about his studies. Sidney began college at Washington University in 1941, and entered the accelerated medical school program at Washington University, receiving his medical degree in 1947. He had finally become a serious scholar, and his parents had another son of whom to be proud.

Research has always been a driving passion in Dr. Goldring's life. During medical school he worked in the lab of Dr. Carl Harford, investigating the etiology of decreased cerebrospinal fluid glucose levels in meningitis, nurturing an early interest in the nervous system. His love of basic research continues today as he surrounds himself with anatomists, physiologists, and engineers working in his neurosurgery department, and he often encourages medical students and residents to consider working on doctorates in basic science.

During medical school Dr. Goldring's interest in the nervous system and the challenges of the developing specialty of neurosurgery confirmed his desire to enter this field. He did his internship and a year of residency in general surgery at the Jewish Hospital in St. Louis. In 1949, he became a fellow in neurology at Washington University working with Dr. James O'Leary. During this time he received his initial training in neurophysiology. In the laboratory he also came under the influence of the inquiring mind of Dr. George Bishop, one of the pioneers in the development of modern neurophysiology. Among Dr. Bishop's many achievements was the first recording of evoked potentials in experimental animals. Dr. Goldring was influenced not only by the scientific achievement of these men, but also by their strong moral character and sense of fairness, the same characteristics that today's generation sees in Dr. Goldring. His life-long interest and understanding in treating patients with severe seizure disorders began at this time, when every morning was spent reading electroencephalograms (EEG) with Dr. O'Leary.

He began his neurosurgery training at Washington University and Barnes Hospital with Dr. Henry Schwartz in 1951. The influence of this superb surgeon and powerful personality has been a guiding force throughout Dr. Goldring's career. His residency was interrupted by 8 months service in the United States Public Health Service as an instructor in neurosurgery with the Washington University Medical Unit in Thailand, an exchange program set up between Washington University and Chulalonkorn and Siriraj Universities in Bangkok. During this time Dr. Goldberg performed the first craniotomy for tumor ever done in Thailand. Returning home, Dr. Goldring entered the United States Army, spending 1 year at Walter Reed Hospital where he first met a future long-time associate, Dr. William Coxe, and worked with Dr. Ludwig Kempe. Dr. Goldring returned to St. Louis and finished his neurosurgical residency at Barnes Hospital in 1956.

Having completed his training Dr. Goldring became a member of the Washington University School of Medicine faculty from 1956 to 1964. He then left Washington University to become professor and head of neurological surgery at the University of Pittsburgh. In 1966, he rejoined Washington University as professor of neurological surgery. When a search committee was formed to find a new head of neurological surgery to replace Dr. Henry Schwartz, the proverbial "legend in his own time," the job seemed herculean; but the answer kept coming back from all sources: "the best man is right there—search no further." In 1974, Dr. Goldring became head of neurological surgery and co-chairman of the newly created Department of Neurology and Neurological Surgery at Washington University School of Medicine, and neurosurgeon-in-chief at Barnes Hospital and St. Louis Children's Hospital. Dr. Goldring has continued the highly respected training program at Washington University in the tradition of Ernest Sachs and Henry Schwartz, encouraging and training neurosurgeons with a strong academic emphasis. In 1980, he was also appointed director of the McDonnell Center for Studies of Higher Brain Function which was created with a large gift from the James S. McDonnell Foundation.

Dr. Goldring's research interests are in neurophysiology and experimental and clinical epilepsy. He has published extensively on these subjects and has developed a large experience in the surgical treatment of seizure disorders. Basic laboratory studies have focused on the steady voltage gradients that exist between the brain and an extracerebral reference, or across the cerebral cortex. These gradients (direct current [DC] potentials) were extensively studied during anoxia, asphyxia, hypoglycemia, focal brain injury, cerebral ischemia, anesthesia, and seizure discharge. Changes in DC potentials were shown to be due to sustained changes in the resting membrane potentials (RMP) of both neurons and glia; the RMP of glia reflecting fluxes in the extracellular K^+ concentration. The glial contribution of these potentials was definitively proven by simultaneous physiologic-morphologic studies in which the glial cells were marked intracellularly with horseradish peroxidase. Clinical research has dealt primarily with epilepsy. His most significant clinical contribution has been the development of a surgical method of treatment in which all surgical manipulation is carried out under general, rather than local, anesthesia. The sensori-motor region is identified in the anesthetized patient by recording cortical sensory evoked responses, and the epileptogenic focus is localized by the use of indwelling surface epidural electrode arrays for extra-operative electrocorticography which is carried out predominantly during spontaneously occurring seizures. This method has made it possible to extend surgical treatment of intractable seizure disorders to patients who heretofore could not as readily be considered for surgery, especially children.

Dr. Goldring has willingly given his time serving the National Institutes of Health and organized neurosurgery. He was a member of the Neurology Study Section of NINCDS from 1964 to 1968 and again from 1969 through 1973, serving as chairman of this section from 1972 to 1973. He was a member of the National Advisory Council of NINCDS from 1977 through 1981. Dr. Goldring was a member of the American Board of Neurological Surgery from 1971 through 1976, serving as chairman from 1974 through 1976. He was chairman of the Residency Review Committee for Neurosurgery from 1974 through 1976.

In 1975, he was chairman of the Neurosciences Interdisciplinary Cluster of the President's Panel on Biomedical and Behavior Research. Currently he is chairman of the Scientific Advisory Committee for the Research Foundation of the American Association of Neurological Surgery (AANS) and has served since 1972, as a member of the Board of Trustees of the Grass Foundation. Dr. Goldring served as president of the Society of Neurological Surgeons from 1981 to 1982, the American Academy of Neurological Surgery from 1982 to 1983, and the AANS from 1984 to 1985.

Sidney Goldring met Lois Blustein when she was 15 years old. Showing characteristic good judgment, he fell in love with this young, beautiful redhead and married her in 1945, when she was a Washington University freshman. A lovely, vibrant, and outgoing woman, Lois has served as a strong complement to Sid while maintaining her own identity in important civic and cultural activities. The Goldrings have two children, James M. Goldring, who in 1985 was a student at the Washington University School of Medicine and completed a Ph.D. in neurobiology before entering medical school, and a daughter, Kathryn Goldring Coryell, who in 1985 lived in Iowa City, Iowa, with her psychiatrist husband, Bill, and children Matthew, then aged 5, and Julie, then aged 1, the special pride of grandparents Lois and Sid. This busy man has little time for hobbies, but vacation time usually finds Sidney and Lois waist deep in the best trout streams of Montana, and a hefty portion of Montana trout find their way to St. Louis deliciously prepared on the table for lucky family and friends.

The Congress of Neurological Surgeons was privileged to recognize Sidney Goldring as its honored guest in 1985.

Robert A. Ratcheson

Robert A. Ratcheson was born in Chicago, Illinois on August 24, 1940. He attended Miami University in Oxford, Ohio and received a B.S. degree from Northwestern University in 1962 and a M.D. degree from Northwestern University School of Medicine in 1965. He served an internship at The Johns Hopkins Hospital and also took a year of general surgery training at that institution. From 1967 to 1969, he was a clinical associate at the National Institutes of Health-Surgical Neurology Branch. Residency training was with Henry G. Schwartz at Barnes Hospital in St. Louis, Missouri. After completion of his residency in 1972, Dr. Ratcheson was a William P. Van Wagenen fellow of the American Association of Neurological Surgeons. He spent a year in the brain research laboratory at Lund University with Dr. Bo K. Siesjo. He was assistant professor of neurological surgery at Washington University from 1973 to 1977 and associate professor from 1977 until 1981. He recalls with gratitude his time at Washington University and the influence of Drs. Henry Schwartz, Sidney Goldring, and William Coxe. In 1981 he was appointed Harvey Huntington Brown, Jr. Professor of Neurological Surgery and chief of the Division of Neurological Surgery at Case Western Reserve University Medical School and Director of Neurological Surgery at University Hospitals of Cleveland. He was greatly influenced during this period by Dr. Frank Nulsen, the previous chief at Case Western Reserve.

During his tenure as president of the Congress of Neurological Surgeons (CNS), Dr. Ratcheson attempted to address the educational mission of the organization. He, with Dr. Fremont P. Wirth, was responsible for the development of the publication, *Concepts in Neurosurgery* and during Dr. Ratcheson's term of office, the Professional Conduct Committee of the Congress was established. Of great importance to him were the close and lasting personal relationships which grew from the professional activities on the CNS Executive Committee. Dr. Ratcheson is a member of a number of medical societies and has served as chairman of the Joint Committee on Education of the American Association of Neurological Surgeons and the Congress of Neurological Surgeons (1985–1988) and is a member of the Board of Directors of the American Board of Neurological Surgery. He has served as a chairman of the Cerebrovascular Surgery Section of the American Association of Neurological Surgeons and the Congress of Neurological Surgeons (1989–1990) and is the current chairman of the Society of Neurological Surgeons' Neurosurgical Committee for Resident Selection and Evaluation. Dr. Ratcheson is a member of the National Advisory Council on Neurological Disorders and Stroke of the National Institutes of Health and of the American Heart Association. He has served on a number of editorial boards, including *Neurosurgery*, and is a member of Alpha Omega Alpha.

His major research interests are in cerebral blood flow and metabolism and various states of neuronal injury. His bibliography lists 63 scientific publications and book chapters. His major clinical interests are in cerebrovascular disease and benign basal skull tumors. More recently, Dr. Ratcheson has served as chairman of the newly formed Department of Neurological Surgery at Case Western Reserve University. In 1964, Dr. Ratcheson married Peggy Steiner, who is a cultural anthropologist. They have three children, Alexey Matthew (21), Rachael Elizabeth (17), and Abigail Marjorie (4).

1986

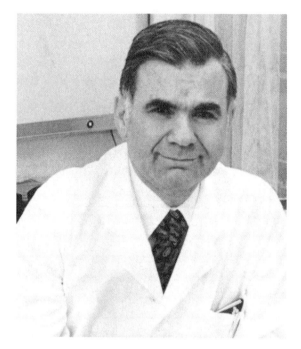

Mahmut Gazi Yasargil

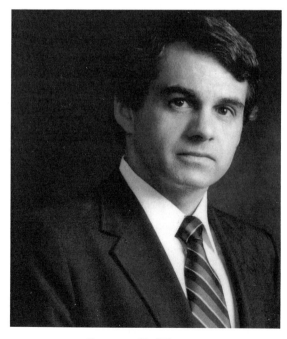

Joseph C. Maroon

Mahmut Gazi Yaşargil

Mahmut Gazi Yasargil was born July 6, 1925, in Lice, a village in eastern Turkey, approximately 200 miles west of the Turko-Iranian border, and 100 miles north of Syria. At the time of Gazi's birth, the population of Lice was 5,000 to 6,000 and the infant mortality rate was about 165 per 1,000 live births. Children were then regarded, particularly among the well educated, as precious assets, to be guarded, guided, loved, and protected. This was certainly true of the two Yasargil sons and daughter. While the family was still young, a move was made to Ankara, partly because of its excellent educational institutions. A tribute to the family's judgment is made by the fact that all three children are quite successful, and two are professors in some branch of medicine in Switzerland today.

Gazi attended Ankara public schools from 1931 to 1943, when he graduated from the Gymnasium. The children were all strongly influenced by their father, who doted on things academic and encouraged the children to work, and to learn from every possible experience. Friends and neighbors of similar background often came to the Yasargil house and carried on spirited discussions on many subjects, including medicine and neurology. At an early age, Gazi became familiar with the terminology of medicine in general and of neurology in particular, as one of Gazi's father's friends was a neurologist.

In 1944, Gazi entered medical school at Frederick Schiller University in Jena, Germany. However, classes were disrupted in 1945 because of World War II and young Gazi transferred to medical school at Basel, Switzerland, where he obtained his medical degree in 1950. Here he was greatly influenced by Professor Muller, a psychiatrist, and his senior thesis was written on the effects of drugs on delirium tremens. This kept Gazi in contact with the principles of cerebral anatomy and physiology, but the concepts of psychiatry were not precise enough for him. His mathematical mind yearned for a problem that he could solve, for a truth which became evident.

In the meantime, Gazi met Professor Hugo Krayenbühl, who headed neurosurgery at the University of Zurich. Young Dr. Yasargil was much impressed by this learned scholar and surgeon, and by the logic and precision of the nervous system. One could localize pathology from a painstaking history of the symptoms and their development, and gain a knowledge of nervous system anatomy and function. Thus, careful examination revealed the location of pathology, while the behavior and pattern of the development of symptoms could reveal the nature of the process. Moreover, if one studied the various tracts of the nervous system, one could determine where along the pathway the process had progressed, and if it were localized or disseminated. It now remained to seek new techniques for examinations that could refine the location of the lesion and perhaps give a clue to its nature.

Gazi joined Dr. Krayenbühl in neurological surgery on January 4, 1953. His admiration for the chief increased, as many facets of care, evaluation, investigation, and theory were revealed to him. Near this same time, a new technique, stereotactic surgery, made its debut. Deep brain lesions were approached without direct vision, by advancing a slender instrument along a set of coordinates, until one reached the site of the problem. Gazi expressed an interest in stereotactic surgery, and he was dispatched to Germany to learn the technique. He found, however, that it was ideal for destroying a given area or a sharply localized lesion, but was not of great value in the repair or reconstruction of tissues.

This was somewhat of a disquieting revelation to Gazi, as his interest at that time was focused on vascular lesions such as aneurysms and arteriovenous malformations. Arteriography, the x-ray technique developed by Lima and Moniz in Portugal, was of greater interest to Gazi, as it actually allowed one to see blood vessels and their exact location. One could now tell whether a vessel required occlusion or repair. For the first time, one could study the angiograms and devise a more precise and physiologically sound operation for ligation or coating of various lesions.

After overcoming the irritating effects of the contrast agents used in arteriography, experience with vascular lesions grew, revealing many problems. One actually needed to count the vessels entering a malformation or aneurysm, and to note the borders of the vessels, so one could recognize them during surgery. The vessels thus identified were often small and their exploration might lead to disruption and bleeding.

New methodology, however, was developing that held some promise. The technique of microsurgery allowed the surgeon to see, by using a dissecting microscope, the lesion in magnified form. The surgery of such fine structures was being studied in the United States, and Gazi was interested. After conveying his interest to Dr. Krayenbühl, an arrangement was made with the Microvascular Laboratory at the University of Vermont, in Burlington, for Dr. Yasargil to join the research staff, where he worked from October 25, 1965 to January 4, 1967. Gazi entered the work wholeheartedly, beginning on the fundamentals, as he wished to miss nothing. In 6 weeks, he finished the exercises customarily performed by a student in 3 months, and was ready for that for which he had come—experience in the handling of the living, functional cortical vessels. This included the direct opening, closing, patching, and surface grafting of the cortical vessels. In essence, Gazi repeated the whole extensive experience that had first been tried on extremities and intraabdominal vessels. However, the vessels Gazi worked with were only 0.5 to 2.0 mm in size!

This remarkable surgeon did not complain about working on the simple problems or that he was ready for the complex. Instead, he studied the available literature and only when he had mastered that knowledge did he plan the research beyond that point. Thus, Gazi gradually decreased the problems to be studied. After just improving the technique of coagulating the small cortical branches that had to be sacrificed, he worked hard and long on preserving every salvageable branch.

A method was sought to allow a vessel (superficial temporal complex) to be grafted into the cortical branch (middle cerebral complex) of the brain. A study of grafts, patch grafts, and replacement grafts had previously been performed with unacceptable failure rates. Gazi conceived of the idea of using the superficial temporal artery as a direct connection into a middle cerebral branch that did not entail the removal of a segment of the superficial temporal artery, and hence did not require a double suture line. The superficial temporal vessel was simply sectioned far enough out to allow it to be sutured to the middle cerebral branch by a single end-to-side anastomosis. This technique provided a greatly improved patency rate and the results were reported in 1967.

Neurosurgeons are familiar with these techniques and with the recent Bypass Study. Under the rules of the study, the procedure was shown not to be helpful in altering mortality and morbidity rates. To give meaning to our data, a study of the physics and physiology of the nervous system blood supply should now be planned.

Perhaps Gazi's greatest contribution to neurosurgery has been his deep and thoughtful study of the subarachnoid spaces. We have all known that careful intracranial operations have low mortality and morbidity rates, provided the brain and its vessels are not injured. What Gazi has done is to demonstrate that many, if not most, intracranial procedures can be done in the subarachnoid space with an intact pia and arachnoid. The problem is that the depths of the wound are sometimes great, the light is poor, and one cannot always be certain where the arachnoid leaves off and the vascular surface remains. Great familiarity with the tissue is needed, and having been there, 10, 20, or 100 times before, is of great importance. Using this knowledge, he has achieved exceedingly low mortality and morbidity rates.

Certainly neurosurgery owes a tremendous debt to the fertile, busy mind of this experienced pioneer. We shall not often see its like. I am grateful to Gazi for what he has taught me. We should all be grateful for what he has taught any of us willing to listen. Mostly we should be grateful on behalf of the thousands of our patients for his demonstration that, with devotion and personal sacrifice, modern neurosurgical procedures can safely be performed.

Yes, the village of Lice is famous for two things: it is the birthplace of Mahmut Gazi Yasargil, and, too, it is the site of a great earthquake. We do not have incontrovertible evidence as to what was cause and what was effect.

R. M. PEARDON DONAGHY, M.D.

Joseph C. Maroon

Dr. Maroon was born in Bridgeport, Ohio, a small coal mining community in the upper Ohio Valley. During his early school years, he excelled in both scholastics and athletics. As a member of the All-Ohio football and baseball first teams, he also was awarded the Coca-Cola Award as an outstanding scholar athlete. He attended Indiana University on an athletic scholarship and was selected as a scholastic All-American in football. He attended Indiana University Medical School and was president of his graduating class. Neurosurgical training was obtained at Georgetown, Indiana, Oxford University in England, and the University of Vermont. After completion of his neurosurgical training, he joined the University of Pittsburgh faculty in 1972 and rose through the ranks to be a professor of neurosurgery. In 1986 he was president of the Congress and it was during that year that the National Think First Program was initiated. In 1984 he became chairman of the Department of Neurological Surgery at Allegheny General Hospital in Pittsburgh and professor of Neurosurgery at the Medical College of Pennsylvania and the University of West Virginia Medical Center. Dr. Maroon has published over 170 papers, 22 chapters, and 1 book. His contributions include the introduction of Doppler ultrasound for the detection of air embolism, the introduction of the Nucleatome for percutaneous discectomy, new surgical techniques for the removal of orbital tumors, and various observations relative to athletic and spinal cord injuries.

1987

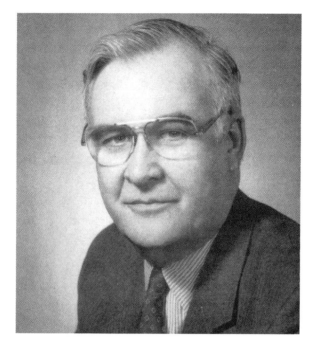

THOMAS WILLIAM LANGFITT

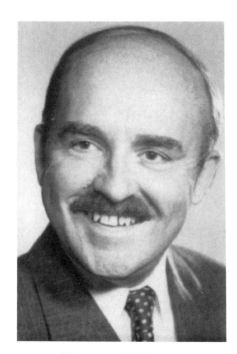

DONALD O. QUEST

Thomas William Langfitt

Thomas William Langfitt was born on April 20, 1927, in Clarksburg, West Virginia, the son of Dr. Frank V. Langfitt and Veda Davis Langfitt. Dr. Frank Langfitt was a general surgeon and an outstanding leader in his community. He played a major role in the creation of the West Virginia University Medical Center in Morgantown and his career and ideals proved to be of great influence on his son's life. Both parents bestowed the values of honesty and integrity upon their son at an early age, attributes for which he is well known and respected.

Dr. Thomas Langfitt graduated from Mercerberg Academy in 1945 and from Princeton University in 1949. He attended The Johns Hopkins Medical School, graduating in 1953. Dr. Langfitt spent many long hours in the library absorbing the fundamentals of medical knowledge and building the intellectual foundation for his investigative life. In addition he got to know the librarian well—Carolyn Louise Payne. They were married in his senior year of medical school. She is the mother of their four sons and continues to be his partner in many civic activities.

Dr. Langfitt completed a tour of duty in the United States Army and returned to The Johns Hopkins for his residency in neurological surgery under Dr. A. Earl Walker. He completed his training in 1961 and moved to Philadelphia, accepting the position of head of the Section of Neurological Surgery at the Pennsylvania Hospital with an academic appointment at the University of Pennsylvania Medical School. Here during the next 7 years he conducted basic research on intracranial pressure, cerebral circulation, and cerebral metabolism.

Continuing his research throughout his long career in neurosurgery, Dr. Langfitt and his colleagues have made major contributions to our understanding of the dynamics and relationships of intracranial pressure, cerebral circulation, and metabolism.

In 1968 he became professor and chairman of the Division of Neurological Surgery at the University of Pennsylvania, a position he held until 1987. He has served as vice president for health affairs at the University and was for a time acting vice president for Finance. Nationally, he has served on numerous advisory councils and committees for the National Institutes of Health. He has been chairman of the Board of the Association of Academic Health Centers and has served as chairman of the Organizing Committee for the International Symposia on Increased Intracranial Pressure and Cerebral Blood Flow. He is a member of the Institute of Medicine of the National Academy of Sciences and is an Honorary Fellow of the Royal College of Surgeons of Edinburgh.

He has served our specialty on the American Board of Neurological Surgery and has been its chairman. He has been on the Board of Directors of the American Association of Neurological Surgeons and has been its vice president. He has been chairman of the Editorial Board of the *Journal of Neurosurgery*, president of the American Academy of Neurological Surgery, and in 1987 was president of the Society of Neurological Surgeons. He has served on the Board of Trustees of Princeton University.

Dr. Langfitt has an impressive bibliography covering many areas of research, both basic and clinical. He has received recognition and honors throughout the world for his scholarly research, his inspired teaching, and his articulate and thoughtful leadership. Literature and the arts are avocations for him and Carolyn and personal physical fitness is high on his list of priorities. He is truly a man for all seasons.

For many years Dr. Langfitt has served on the Board of Directors of the Glenmede Trust Company, the administrators of the Pew Charitable Trust. This Trust is the second largest in the United States and provides significant financial support for biomedical research and projects beneficial to society in general. In February 1987, Dr. Langfitt retired as chairman of the Division of Neurological Surgery at the University of Pennsylvania to assume the duties of his new post—president and chief executive officer of the Glenmede Trust Company and Pew Charitable Trust, one more remarkable achievement for this remarkable man.

I am indebted to Dr. Frederick Murtagh, a long-time colleague and friend of Dr. Langfitt's, who wrote his biography in *Surgical Neurology* in 1984. The Congress of Neurological Surgeons was proud to have Dr. Thomas Langfitt as honored guest at its annual meeting in Baltimore in 1987.

DONALD O. QUEST, M.D.

Donald O. Quest

Donald O. Quest was born on November 20, 1939 in St. Louis, Missouri. He graduated from the Riverview Gardens High School in St. Louis in 1957. He graduated with honors from the University of Illinois with a B.S. degree in mathematics in 1961. He served on active duty with the United States Navy as a naval aviator between 1961 and 1966. Don then attended the Columbia University College of Physicians and Surgeons and was awarded an M.D. degree in 1970. He was elected to Alpha Omega Alpha and received the Winchester prize for overall excellence in his graduating medical school class. He interned in surgery at the Massachusetts General Hospital between 1970 and 1971 and then was a resident in surgery from 1971 to 1972. Dr. Quest was a resident in neurological surgery at the Neurological Institute in New York at the Columbia Presbyterian Medical Center between 1972 and 1975. He was chief resident from 1975 to 1976. He served as an assistant professor of neurological surgery at the Downstate Medical Center of the State University of New York between 1976 and 1978. He was appointed instructor in neurological surgery at the Columbia University College of Physicians and Surgeons in 1978, and rose through the ranks to become professor of clinical neurosurgery in 1989.

Dr. Quest served on the Executive Committee of the Congress of Neurological Surgeons from 1978 to 1988. He was chairman of the Scientific Program Committee at the annual meeting in 1982 and was treasurer of the Congress between 1981 and 1984. He was president from 1986 to 1987. The annual meeting in Baltimore in 1987 was a great success.

In addition to the Congress of Neurosurgeons, Dr. Quest is a member of the

American Association of Neurological Surgeons (AANS), the American Academy of Neurological Surgeons, the American College of Surgeons, the American Medical Association, the Neurosurgical Society of America, and the Society of Neurological Surgeons. He is now on the Board of Directors of the American Association of Neurological Surgeons and was chairman of the Scientific Program Committee of the AANS from 1990 to 1991. Dr. Quest has been a visiting professor at many medical centers in the United States and was a visiting professor at the Kyoto Prefecturial University in Kyoto, Japan in 1988. Dr. Quest has a bibliography of 49 papers.

Don Quest married Ilona Madis on July 20, 1969. Dr. and Mrs. Quest have three children, Wendy Elaine, Amy Ilona, and Susan Elissa. Dr. Quest has taken his civic responsibilities very seriously. He has served as president of the Board of Education in HoHoKus, New Jersey from 1983 to 1986 and has worked with numerous other civic and corporate bodies.

1988

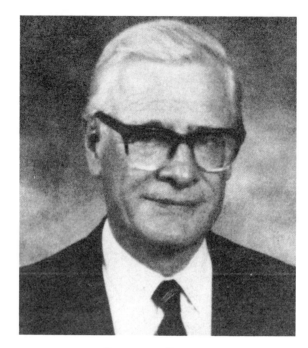

LINDSAY SYMON

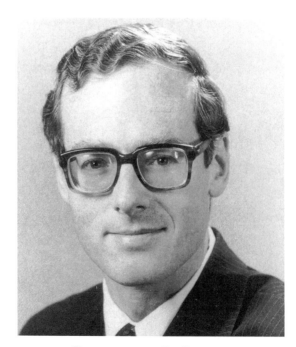

CHRISTOPHER B. SHIELDS

Lindsay Symon

Professor Lindsay Symon, the honored guest of the Congress of Neurological Surgeons (CNS) for 1988, was born in Aberdeen, Scotland, in 1929. He graduated from grammar school and Aberdeen University with outstanding academic achievements, having won virtually every scholastic award offered. His early attraction to the neurosciences was evident on his being awarded the Fulton Prize in Neurology for his dissertation on "The Natural History and Treatment of Migraine." Professor Symon was the outstanding graduate from Aberdeen University in 1951. He obtained his early clinical training in Aberdeen and became a clinical research fellow for the Medical Research Council in Physiology and Pharmacology at the National Institute for Medical Research in London. At the same time, he was also a registrar in neurosurgery at the Middlesex and Maida Vale Hospitals, a dual appointment he has maintained throughout his entire professional career.

In 1961, he was awarded a Rockefeller Traveling Fellowship in Medicine, which he took to Dr. John Sterling Meyer at Wayne State University in Detroit. It was here that he developed a major interest in the cerebral circulation and metabolism, which has remained a major topic of his research endeavors.

He completed his neurosurgical training at the Middlesex and Maida Vale Hospitals in 1968, following which he was appointed consultant to the National Hospitals at Queen's Square and Maida Vale. In 1978, he became professor of neurological surgery and chairman of the Gough Cooper Department of Neurological Surgery at the National Hospital, Queen's Square, in London. There he has developed an outstanding neurosurgical training program, which is considered one of the leading units in England. Research endeavors there have stressed not only his own interests in cerebral circulation and cerebral metabolism but also an active neurooncology laboratory of his associates. Three years ago, he was the recipient of the John Hunter Award of the College of Surgeons of England for research in cerebrovascular disorders. Professor Symon is the first neurosurgeon in the 100-year history of this award to be so honored.

Professor Symon is a prolific writer and has authored or coauthored over 400 publications, monographs, and books. His scientific interests have extended over a broad range of topics, including *Advances and Technical Standards in Neurosurgery* and *Acta Neurochirurgica*. He is a clinical surgeon par excellence, as well as an outstanding teacher and leader of young physicians. His pastimes are traveling and playing his beloved game of golf. He rarely travels to a meeting that he does not play if time allows. As a true connoisseur of the sport, he invariably makes time for it.

His wife, Pauline, frequently accompanies him on his many trips, including this Congress meeting. The Symons have three children. In 1988, their son was a physicist who ran a language school in Osaka, one daughter was an Arabic scholar who was working for the British Broadcasting Corporation, and the other daughter was a physician in Hungerford, England.

Professor Symon was named "Surgeon of the Year" by *Surgical Neurology* in 1985. It was a privilege to have him as the honored guest of the Congress in 1988.

CHRISTOPHER B. SHIELDS, M.D.

Christopher B. Shields

Dr. Shields was the first Canadian president of the Congress. He was born in Schumacher, a small gold-mining town in northern Ontario where he lived until finishing secondary school. He graduated from medical school at the University of Toronto in 1966 and completed his neurosurgical residency in Winnipeg, Canada at the University of Manitoba under the direction of Dwight Parkinson. Following his residency he spent 1 year as a fellow in microvascular neurosurgery at the University of Vermont under Peardon Donaghy. Since 1974, he has spent his entire professional life at the University of Louisville where he is now professor and co-director of the Division of Neurological Surgery, and co-director of the Kenton D. Leatherman Spine Center. He has also served as chairman of the Cerebrovascular Section of the American Association of Neurological Surgeons (AANS) and Congress of Neurological Surgeons (CNS), and as annual meeting chairman of the AANS in 1989. His primary areas of neurosurgical expertise are in spinal surgery and stereotactic radiosurgery with research interests in spinal cord protection and regeneration as well as in developing techniques of intraoperative neuromonitoring. He is married to Deborah Dickson from Winnipeg. They have two daughters, Lisa and Karen, who are accomplished pianists, having won several Kentucky State music competitions, and having competed in Southern regional piano competitions. Lisa will attend Duke University this year and Karen will be a junior in high school.

The 1988 annual meeting of the CNS was held in the Pacific Northwest (Seattle) for the first time which provided the theme for the social events during the week. During the planning stages of the meeting the convention center was still under construction so there was considerable doubt and consternation that it would be completed in time for the meeting. It was finished only 1 month before the meeting date and the Congress was the first major event to be held in the Washington State Convention Trade Center.

The Congress was pleased to have Lindsay Symon as its honored guest in 1988. Professor Symon was the second British neurosurgeon to hold this position. Professor Symon's graciousness and scientific contributions were the highlight of the annual meeting, particularly his valuable advice to the neurosurgical residents. The meeting's major themes were future pathways in health care delivery, spinal surgery, vascular surgery, and glioma surgery. Thomas Saul was the annual meeting chairman and Nick Hopkins served as scientific program chairman. Kim Burchiel was the local arrangements chairman for the beautiful "Emerald City." A postconvention meeting was held in Victoria, Canada at the Princess Hotel, which was attended by more than 200 members. The group enjoyed a 3-hour scenic catamaran ride from Seattle. The postconvention hosts were Barbara and Brian Hunt.

The year 1987 to 1988 marked the creation of the Joint Neurosurgical Task Force on the Decade of the Brain of the CNS/AANS with the charge to create innovative and imaginative ways for neurosurgery to be involved in the congressionally designated Decade of the Brain, 1990 to 2000. The primary goal of the committee, chaired by Dr. Shields, has been to increase public funding of neuroscience research, and to increase the public's awareness of the role played by neurosurgery in the betterment of society. Neurosurgery is acting in cooperation with neurology, the basic neurosciences, and psychiatry in this international project under the umbrella of the National Coalition of Brain Research. Neurosurgery has focused on a specific topic during each year of the decade such as CNS trauma and stroke, brain tumors, the surgical treatment of epilepsy, stereotactic and functional neurosurgery, etc. It is hoped that by using this mechanism, a significant increase of research dollars will become part of the annual National Institutes of Health funding for neurosurgical research.

1989

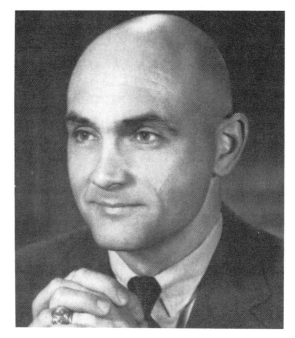

THORALF M. SUNDT, JR.

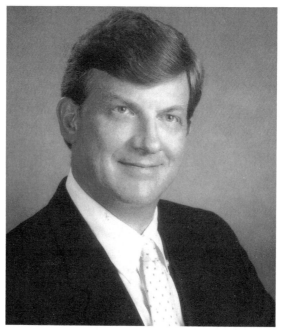

J. MICHAEL MCWHORTER

Thoralf M. Sundt, Jr.

The honored guest for the 1989 meeting of the Congress of Neurological Surgeons was Dr. Thoralf M. Sundt, Jr., chairman of the Department of Neurological Surgery at the Mayo Clinic and professor of Neurological Surgery at the Mayo Medical School. He is an internationally recognized leader in cerebrovascular surgery who has written more than 200 articles on this subject.

Dr. Sundt's initial career interests lay in the military and not in medicine. As the middle son of an architect, he followed in the footsteps of his two uncles and entered the United States Military Academy at West Point at the age of 18 years. After graduation, he had a distinguished career in the Korean War and was awarded the Bronze Star with Oak Leaf Cluster.

Because "practicing for war was boring," he decided to pursue a career in medicine and subsequently entered the University of Tennessee Medical School in 1956. Inspired by Dr. Eustace Semmes and Dr. Francis Murphey, he undertook his residency training at the University of Tennessee. During his residency, he spent 6 months at the Mayo Clinic studying medical neurology. Impressed by the large number of surgical cases done there and the opportunity to work with Dr. Collin MacCarty and Dr. Ross Miller, he returned to the Mayo Clinic upon completion of his residency for additional training. His interest in cerebrovascular surgery developed while working in the laboratory with Dr. Arthur G. Waltz. During this period, his concern for the high morbidity and mortality related to direct surgical approaches to intracranial aneurysms stimulated the development of the encircling clip grafts for aneurysms that tear at their base.

In 1966, he joined the University of Tennessee faculty and in 3 years operated on more than 150 intracranial aneurysms. In 1969, he was offered a staff position at the Mayo Clinic. Since then, he has refined surgical techniques for operations such as carotid endarterectomy and intracranial aneurysms with results considered among the best in neurosurgery. He continues to recognize the role of revascularization procedures for cerebral ischemia.

Dr. Sundt has been an active participant in organized neurosurgery. He is currently the editor of the *Journal of Neurosurgery*. In 1989, he held the chairmanship of the Credentials Committee of the American Board of Neurological Surgery and was president of the American Academy of Neurological Surgeons. In 1991, Dr. Sundt was inducted into the Institute of Medicine of the National Academy of Sciences.

His professional successes have been transcended by his role as husband and father. The faithful and loving support of his wife, Lois, has been a mainstay for 36 years. Their three children are Laura, a successful businesswoman; Thoralf, who is completing his training in cardiac surgery; and John, an attorney. Dr. Sundt's hobbies and interests include military history, violin, ecology, and arboreal horticulture.

Dr. Sundt is highly respected and admired by his colleagues as a skilled neurosurgeon and a gentleman. Among those he has trained, he enjoys the deepest loyalty and esteem.

PHILIP W. TALLY, M.D.

J. Michael McWhorter

J. Michael McWhorter was born in Hattiesburg, Mississippi on November 8, 1941. He was awarded a B.S. degree from the University of Southern Mississippi in Hattiesburg in 1963. He graduated from the University of Mississippi School of Medicine in 1968. He interned at the North Carolina Baptist Hospital from 1968 to 1969 and started his residency there. His training was interrupted by 2 years of active duty with the United States Navy between 1970 and 1972. He rose to the rank of lieutenant commander and served on the USS *Guadalcanal*.

Dr. McWhorter returned to the North Carolina Baptist Hospital where he was a resident in neurological surgery between 1972 and 1977. During this time he served a fellowship in neuropathology and also a fellowship in neurology. He was a fellow in microneurosurgery at the Christ Hospital Institute of Medical Research in Cincinnati from January to June of 1976 and then was a fellow in microneurosurgery in Zurich, Switzerland in 1976. Dr. McWhorter was invited to join the faculty of neurosurgery at Bowman Gray School of Medicine in 1977. He started out as an instructor and is now an associate professor.

Dr. McWhorter became very active in the Congress of Neurological Surgeons. He was the annual meeting chairman for the meeting in New Orleans in 1986 and was president at the 1989 meeting in Atlanta with Dr. Thoralf M. Sundt, Jr. as the honored guest. Dr. McWhorter has been very interested in international neurological surgery. He was a member of a visiting surgical team in St. Croix, Virgin Islands in 1979 and in Haiti in 1980. He was a visiting faculty member at the Tokai University Hospital in Japan in March 1990.

Dr. McWhorter has been very busy in the clinical practice of neurological surgery, teaching, and research. However, he has not forgotten that medicine is only part of the larger world and he is an active member of the Rotary Club of Winston-Salem. His teacher, and former chief and honored guest in 1980, Dr. Eben Alexander, Jr., was a former president of the same Rotary Club. Dr. McWhorter has served on the Board of Directors of the Rotary Club from 1983 to the present. He has served on the Venture-in-Mission Committee of the Episcopal Diocese of North Carolina and on the Board of Deacons of the Knollwood Baptist Church from 1984 to 1992. He served on the Board of Directors of the Forsyth-Stokes Mental Health Authority in 1984. Dr. McWhorter married Barbara Dix and they have three children, two daughters and a son.

1990

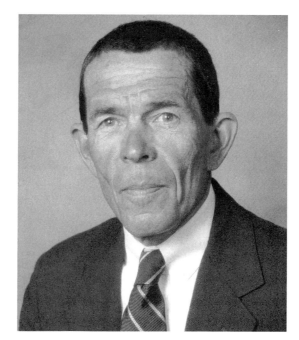

CHARLES BYRON WILSON

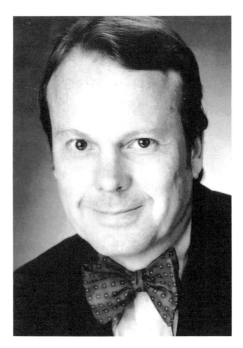

HAL LOMAX HANKINSON

Charles Byron Wilson

Charles Byron Wilson was born August 31, 1929, in Neosho, Missouri in the heart of the Ozarks. Known as the City of Flowers, Neosho (pop. 5000) was featured in Life Magazine as a typical 1940s American small town. Dr. Wilson's father was a druggist and an important member of the community.

As a young man, Dr. Wilson was influenced by a Tulane alumnus living in Neosho, and went to New Orleans on a football scholarship, planning to enter either medicine or the ministry. His career as a halfback was relatively short-lived and he settled on medicine, graduating first in his class in 1954. George Burch, the esteemed cardiologist, nearly convinced Dr. Wilson to go into internal medicine. Dr. Wilson took a rotating internship and 1 year in pathology at Charity Hospital, finding neuropathology, neurology, and neuroanatomy fascinating. He was drawn to neurosurgery by Dr. Dean Echols, the respected mentor of many Tulane neurosurgeons. During his time in New Orleans, Dr. Wilson was able to put his musical talent to work playing the piano in the French Quarter.

After completing his residency at Tulane, he joined the faculty briefly before becoming assistant professor of neurosurgery at Louisiana State University Medical School from 1961 to 1963, and won the Best Teacher Award in 1963. That same year he moved to Lexington and established the Division of Neurosurgery at the University of Kentucky. While there, he pursued his increasing interest in malignant gliomas and developed laboratory and clinical research programs. He received both the Outstanding Clinical Instructor and Outstanding Clinical Professor awards at Kentucky. He then was named professor and chairman of the Division of Neurosurgery at the University of California, San Francisco in 1968, and established the internationally respected Department of Neurosurgery there in 1970. He has been Tong-Po Kan Professor of Neurosurgery since 1985.

Doctor Wilson has expertise and extensive experience in many facets of neurosurgery, and has a special interest in pituitary disorders, having performed more than 2,000 transsphenoidal operations. Aneurysms, particularly of the posterior circulation, and the cervical spine also are areas of particular interest. However, Dr. Wilson justifiably is most proud of his accomplishments related to the establishment of the Brain Tumor Research Center at UCSF, which not only treats over 4,500 brain tumor patients each year, but also has contributed extensively to basic and applied research in neurooncology.

He has received numerous awards and honors and has been the Wilder Penfield Lecturer, the Herbert Olivecrona Lecturer, and the R. Eustace Semmes Lecturer among others. He has published more than 500 articles and chapters and has served on numerous editorial boards, including that of the *Journal of Neurosurgery* which he chaired from 1981 to 1983.

Dr. Wilson is a charismatic, scholarly, dedicated, and energetic leader and surgeon. He has contributed significantly to medical science and trained a growing number of neurosurgeons who are continuing his tradition of excellence in patient care and investigation of nervous system disorders. We were delighted to have him as honored guest for the Congress of Neurological Surgeons annual meeting in Los Angeles, in 1990.

HAL LOMAX HANKINSON, M.D.

Hal Lomax Hankinson

Hal Lomax Hankinson was born in Tyler, Texas, on December 23, 1942. His father was in the oil business and ultimately the family moved to Houston where Hal attended high school. He became interested in the biological sciences while attending the University of Texas in Austin, from which he graduated in 1963, with a B.A. degree in biology *cum laude*. His medical school years were spent in New Orleans at Tulane. There he was elected to Alpha Omega Alpha in his junior year and graduated first in the class of 1967. Internship was in surgery at the Charity Hospital of Louisiana. Dr. Hankinson served in the Navy as a submarine medical officer. In 1970, he began his residency at the University of California, San Francisco under Chairman Charles B. Wilson. In 1972, he married Donna Cameron, and following the completion of formal training, the couple moved to Albuquerque, New Mexico, where Dr. Hankinson has practiced private neurosurgery for 16 years. Shortly after moving to Albuquerque, the first of their two children was born. Dr. Hankinson became involved in the Congress of Neurological Surgeons in 1975 and was given his first major task as sergeant-at-arms chairman. He then served on the Executive Committee, was treasurer and vice president before being selected as president elect in 1988. The 1990 meeting was held in Los Angeles at the Century Plaza Hotel. Doctor Hankinson's presidential address was entitled "Privilege and Obligation" and emphasized the positive aspects of practicing neurosurgery during changing times.

Dr. Hankinson practices general neurosurgery with a special interest in skull base surgery and is on the staff of several hospitals in Albuquerque. He is a clinical professor of neurosurgery at the University of New Mexico.

1991

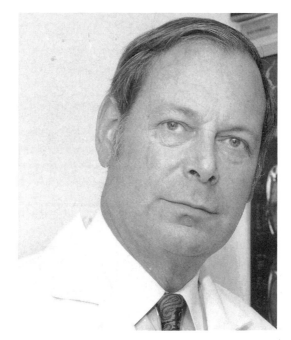

Bennett Mueller Stein

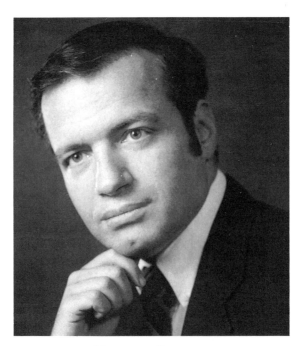

Michael Salcman

Bennett Mueller Stein

Bennett Mueller Stein is a man of many talents spanning neurosurgery, teaching, research, scholarship, athletics, and auto mechanics. The single element common to all these seemingly unrelated endeavors is the pursuit of excellence, which has fostered his continued growth and made his accomplishments the standards by which subsequent achievements are measured.

Born February 2, 1931 in New York City, New York, Ben grew up in Cliffside Park and Ridgefield, New Jersey where he attended public school. As an only child, he was extremely close to his immediate and distant relatives, and family remains one of his highest priorities.

The influence of his parents was especially significant. His father, Walter, held an engineering degree and for many years worked for General Electric. In later years, he and his brother, Albert, purchased and ran a local newspaper, *The Palisadian*. Ben grew up watching his father work on mechanical projects at home, and it was during this time that he developed his enduring fascination with cars and clocks. It is not difficult to trace the origins of his delight in precise and intricate problem-solving.

His mother, Marjorie, was an English teacher in Cliffside Park, a professional woman at a time when career mothers were rare. Her emphasis on education, achievement, and a high quality of performance certainly helped shape Ben's standards and career goals.

Two vignettes from childhood summers at the family lake house in New Jersey illustrate the development of Ben's curiosity about how things worked and his business acumen. He persuaded his father to place an advertisement in the local newspaper for someone to sit in the refrigerator and determine whether the light actually did go off when the door was closed! A few years later, he and a friend formed a salvage company and, for a modest fee, they would search the bottom of the lake for lost items.

When he graduated from Dwight-Morrow High School in 1948, Ben intended to pursue a career in engineering and his college choices were between Rensslaer Polytechnic Institute and Dartmouth College. His mother, in a prescient moment, handed him an issue of *Parade Magazine* and said, "You should be a doctor like this neurosurgeon." The man on the cover was Dr. J. Lawrence Pool and the article discussed his experimental work in psychosurgery. As a first-year resident in 1960, Ben finally met Dr. Pool and, 20 years later, he succeeded his mentor as chief at the Neurological Institute.

However, the choice of neurosurgery did not coincide with the adolescent discovery of a role model. After earning an A.B. degree from Dartmouth in 1952, Ben began the 2-year Dartmouth medical course which, because of the teaching method, did not appeal to his love of order and logic. Fortunately, during the second year, he observed Dr. Robert Fisher, a neurosurgeon in the college clinic. Suddenly, neurosurgery as an academic discipline and a lifelong career choice became very exciting, and his course was firmly established.

The final years of medical school were taken at McGill University where Ben attained his M.D. in 1955, followed by a rotating internship at the United States Naval Hospital, St. Albans, New York. Between 1956 and 1958, he fulfilled his military obligation on the neurological services in the United

States Naval Hospitals at Bethesda and Great Lakes. He currently holds the rank of Lt. Commander USNR-MC, Ret. From 1958 to 1959, Ben was a Fulbright scholar at the National Hospital in Queen's Square, London.

Upon his return, Ben took a year of assistant general surgical residency at Presbyterian Hospital, and then 4 years of neurosurgical residency at the Neurological Institute. By 1962 his earliest publications (with W. F. McCormick) were already devoted to vascular diseases. After completion of his residency, Ben became a special fellow of the NINDB in neuroanatomy and studied with Malcolm Carpenter at Columbia University. Published investigations on the vestibular nuclei, subthalamus, and dorsal roots of the primate spinal cord soon followed. Together with his mentor, J. Lawrence Pool, and Richard A. Fraser, he published a series of seminal publications on vasospasm and the noradrenergic system. In 1971, he left Columbia to become professor and chairman of neurological surgery at Tufts University School of Medicine in Boston. The same year, his classic paper on the infratentorial supracerebellar approach to pineal lesions was published. While at Tufts, S. M. Wolpert and Ben began their research on combined embolization and excision for the treatment of cerebral arteriovenous malformations (AVM). This work was soon extended to spinal AVMs and Ben became interested in intramedullary spinal cord tumors as well. It is interesting to see how often Ben's earlier investigative work has presaged a subsequent clinical interest. In 1980, he was called back to Columbia to serve as Byron Stookey Professor of Neurological Surgery and chairman of the department at the College of Physicians and Surgeons. In addition to his teaching and administrative responsibilities, Ben has remained extraordinarily productive, having authored more than 170 scientific works and extending his studies of AVMs and pineal region tumors to include the chemical reactivity of vessels and the hormonal activity of tumors.

The desire to excel has characterized all areas of Ben's life. He lettered in track in high school and rowed crew in college. He is an accomplished tennis player and a superb skier. His most passionate avocation, however, is Ben's Motor Service, a professional auto mechanic shop where, with the same elegant precision he brings to neurosurgery, he rebuilds and cares for a fleet of bright red sports cars.

Ben's early devotion to family has deepened and extended to the family he has helped create. While a student at McGill, he met and married Doreen Holmes, a nurse at the University Hospital. They had two daughters, Susan, now married to Alan Bachman, and Marjorie, now married to Warren Marcucci. Several years after Doreen passed away, Ben was fortunate enough to find happiness again when he met and married Bonita Soontit. In 1989, Ben achieved two milestones: he became a grandfather for the first time when Rebecca was born to Marjorie and Warren, and he became a father for the third time when Bennett Charles Stein arrived.

Ben has served as a governor of the American College of Surgeons, on the Executive Committee of the American Academy of Neurological Surgeons, as a director of the American Board of Neurological Surgery, and as treasurer and president of the Society of Neurological Surgeons. To every endeavor, he brings the same thoughtful and deliberate attention to detail that characterizes his meticulous operative technique. His calm manner, love of teaching, and exquisite technique have made him a beloved mentor to residents at two fine institutions. The Congress of Neurological Surgeons is deeply honored to have Bennett M. Stein serve as our honored guest.

Michael Salcman

Michael Salcman was born in Pilsen, Czechoslovakia and came to the United States in 1948. After attending public schools in New York, he entered the 6-year Combined Program in Liberal Arts and Medical Education at Boston University and served a surgical internship at the University Hospital in Boston. He was a fellow in neurophysiology in the Laboratory of Neural Control at the National Institutes of Health and received his training in neurosurgery at the Neurological Institute of Columbia University from 1972 to 1976. Thereafter, he joined the faculty of the University of Maryland School of Medicine where he started the Neuro-Oncology Service and headed the Neuro-Trauma Service at the Maryland Institute for Emergency Medical Services Systems. He became professor and head of the Division of Neurological Surgery in 1983. His clinical research has concentrated on brain tumors of all types, arterio-venous malformations, aneurysms, and head injury. His laboratory research has been devoted to such areas as microwave hyperthermia and cerebral blood flow, the blood-brain barrier, model brain tumors, and the *in vitro* investigation of combined modality therapy. He is the author of more than 160 scientific articles and book chapters as well as two textbooks, one on neurologic emergencies and the other, the neurobiology of brain tumors.

Dr. Salcman has served on numerous Congress committees and as associate editor of *Neurosurgery*. He became secretary of the Congress in 1983 and helped computerize its membership files. He was one of the first to initiate a program of exchange visits between the officers of the Congress and the Japanese Congress of Neurological Surgery. In addition to international affairs and technology, Dr. Salcman has emphasized the educational and humanitarian thrust of the organization. As president, he has worked intensively with the Think First Foundation, on the Decade of the Brain project, and with the Washington Committee.

Dr. Salcman became president in 1990 and during his tenure, international membership was increased and the benefits of such membership expanded. In addition, a committee was appointed to develop neurosurgical humanitarian efforts in the Third World. Together with the Washington Committee and other leaders, Dr. Salcman worked to set the scientific agenda for the Decade of the Brain in regard to National Institutes of Health appropriations. He also helped provide Congress input into the financial aspects of health care delivery. Both as president and as chairman of the Joint Committee on Education, he has worked to strengthen the commitment of organized neurosurgery to continuing medical education. The publication of an official history of the Congress is the culmination of a dream that he has shared with several other presidents.

His interests outside the Congress and neurosurgery include his family, sailing, scuba diving, poetry, and contemporary art. Dr. Salcman has served as president of the Friends of Modern Art at the Baltimore Museum of Art and as an active member of the Accessions Committee of its Board of Trustees. He and his wife Ilene have provided numerous art groups from both Washington, D.C. and the Baltimore area with guided tours of their own collection.

Dr. Salcman has served on the Executive Committee of the Congress since 1981 and treasures above all else the friendships of his neurosurgical colleagues.